PINK THERAPY

A guide for therapists working with lesbian, gay and bisexual clients

Edited by
DOMINIC DAVIES
and
CHARLES NEAL

OPEN UNIVERSITY PRESS
Buckingham · Philadelphia

Open University Press
Celtic Court
22 Ballmoor
Buckingham
MK18 1XW

email: enquiries@openup.co.uk
world wide web: www.openup.co.uk

and
325 Chestnut Street
Philadelphia, PA 19106, USA

First Published 1996
Reprinted 1996, 1997, 1999, 2000

Copyright © the editors and contributors 1996

All rights reserved. Except for the quotation of short passages for the purpose of criticism and review, no part of this publication may be reproduced, stored in a retrieval system, or transmitted, in any form or by any means, electronic, mechanical, photocopying, recording or otherwise, without the prior written permission of the publisher or a licence from the Copyright Licensing Agency Limited. Details of such licences (for reprographic reproduction) may be obtained from the Copyright Licensing Agency Ltd of 90 Tottenham Court Road, London, W1P 0LP.

A catalogue record of this book is available from the British Library

ISBN 0 335 19145 2 (pbk)   0 335 19657 8

Library of Congress Cataloging-in-Publication Data
Pink therapy : a guide for counsellors and therapists working with
  lesbian, gay, and bisexual clients / edited by Dominic Davies and
  Charles Neal.
      p. cm.
    Includes bibliographical references and index.
    ISBN 0-335-19657-8. — ISBN 0-335-19145-2 (pbk.)
    1. Gays—Mental health. 2. Bisexuals—Mental health. 3. Gays—
  Counselling of. 4. Bisexuals—Counselling of. I. Davies, Dominic,
  1959-   . II. Neal, Charles, therapist.
  RC451.4.G39P54   1996   95-26372
  616.89´008´664—dc20   CIP

Typeset by Graphicraft Typesetters Ltd, Hong Kong
Printed in Great Britain by Biddles Limited, www.biddles.co.uk

This book is dedicated to all those who are prepared to work to alleviate the isolation and oppression of lesbian, gay and bisexual people. It is our hope that through this book lesbian, gay and bisexual clients and therapists will no longer need to take the responsibility to educate and inform heterosexual therapists of the diversity of our culture and lifestyles and the importance of our therapeutic equality.

Contents

Dedication	iii
Notes on contributors	vii
Acknowledgements	ix
Introduction *Charles Neal and Dominic Davies*	1

PART I: Fundamental issues

1	An historical overview of homosexuality and therapy *Dominic Davies with Charles Neal*	11
2	Towards a model of gay affirmative therapy *Dominic Davies*	24
3	Homophobia and heterosexism *Dominic Davies*	41
4	Working with people coming out *Dominic Davies*	66

PART II: Working with particular issues

5	Working with single people *Lyndsey Moon*	89
6	Working with people in relationships *Gail Simon*	101

7	Lesbian and gay parenting issues *Helena Hargaden and Sara Llewellin*	116
8	Working with young people *Dominic Davies*	131
9	Working with older lesbians *Val Young*	149
10	Working with older gay men *Bernard Ratigan*	159
11	Alcohol and substance misuse *Graz Kowszun and Maeve Malley*	170
12	Partner abuse *Fran Walsh*	188
13	Religious and spirituality conflicts *Bernard Lynch*	199

Appendix 1 Resources 209
Appendix 2 Community resources 213
Appendix 3 Books for clients and counsellors 217

References 222
Index 235

Notes on contributors

Dominic Davies has a wide experience of 'people work' in the statutory and voluntary sectors. He is currently senior lecturer in counselling at the Nottingham Trent University. He has previously worked in university counselling and as a training consultant in HIV/AIDS work and sexuality issues. He runs an independent practice supervising and providing therapy. He holds a diploma in person-centred counselling and psychotherapy, is a BAC-accredited counsellor and co-chair of the Association for Lesbian, Gay and Bisexual Psychologies (UK Section).

Helena Hargaden is a UKCP-registered psychotherapist and BAC-accredited counsellor. Helena practises therapy and supervision in London and teaches counsellors and therapists. She identifies as a bisexual woman currently raising two sons born into her committed relationship with Sara Llewellin.

Graz Kowszun is a BAC-accredited counsellor in private practice, a supervisor and counsellor trainer at Morley and Lewisham Colleges. Having worked for over a decade in the alcohol, drugs and HIV fields, she is consolidating her humanistic integrative approach through psychotherapy training at metanoia in London.

Sara Llewellin is in advanced training in transactional analysis at metanoia. She directs a voluntary sector organization and came out as a teenager. She has been involved in raising children ever since. She is raising two sons born into her committed relationship with her partner Helena Hargaden.

Dr Bernard Lynch is a Roman Catholic priest with an interdisciplinary doctorate in theology and psychology, and works in New York and the UK. He has been the subject of three documentaries on Channel Four and is author of the book *Priest on Trial* (Bloomsbury 1993). He is a member of the Mayor of New York's Task Force on AIDS.

Maeve Malley trained at City University, Kent University, Women's Therapy Centre and the Institute of Family Therapy. Currently senior counsellor at Newham Alcohol Advisory Service in East London, she is particularly interested in working with lesbians and women generally around dependency issues.

Lyndsey Moon is presently studying for a PhD at Essex University focusing on the role of counselling with lesbian, gay and bisexual clients. She gained a BSc in psychology and an MSc in counselling from Goldsmiths College, University of London. She also works as a counsellor in private practice in northwest London.

Charles Neal is a therapist, trainer and educator with 25 years' experience working towards empowerment with people of all ages at points of change. He specializes in gay affirmative therapy and working with artists and performers. Co-parenting two sons with his partner Jeremy has been a rich and wonderful experience. He is founding chair of the Association for Lesbian, Gay and Bisexual Psychologies in the UK, and a graduate of Spectrum's humanistic and integrative psychotherapy training.

Dr Bernard Ratigan is consultant adult psychotherapist in the Nottingham Psychotherapy Unit and in the Department of Genito-Urinary Medicine, City Hospital, Nottingham. He is a registered psychoanalytic psychotherapist with UKCP, a member of the training committee of the South Trent Training in Dynamic Psychotherapy, an accredited counsellor with BAC and a member of the Association for Lesbian, Gay and Bisexual Psychologies.

Gail Simon works as a counsellor with the Pink Practice, a lesbian and gay counselling service in London. She also teaches psychotherapy, offers consultations and runs support groups for staff teams. Gail has a particular interest in the politics of therapy.

Fran Walsh has a background in the voluntary sector and in mental health. She has worked as a counsellor for nine years and holds a diploma in person-centred counselling and psychotherapy and is in private practice as a therapist and supervisor. She also has a number of years' experience as a training consultant.

Val Young is an able-bodied older lesbian of Indian-British, Jewish and Irish heritage. She is a women's psychotherapist and has done a variety of training work. She is author of *The Equality Complex: Lesbians in Therapy – a Guide to Anti-Oppressive Practice*, a practice text on anti-oppressive therapy (Cassell 1995b).

Acknowledgements

Dominic would like to thank the following people for their help and support in writing and preparing this book:

- My supervisors and trainers who nurtured my interest in the field and offered wise counsel. I began as a precocious young man of 21 years, and have been privileged over the past 14 years to have worked with some of the best therapists in Britain: Michael Jacobs, Moira Walker, Bernard Ratigan, Colin Lago, Brian Thorne, Dave Mearns and Elke Lambers. I am grateful for the opportunity to have them as my teachers.
- Jan Bridget, Angela Cameron, Adrian Coyle, Allan O'Leary, Graham Perlman, Fran Walsh and Zak Webber for their constructive feedback and editorial support, and Alan Frankland – without his constant support and clarity of mind I would have given up on this project long ago.
- The library staff at the University of Nottingham for their efficiency in ordering interlibrary loans and helping me locate obscure books and references.

Charles would like to thank Jeremy Cole, my partner, for his loving patience and support, our two sons Sam and Jago for their indulgence during months of distracted negligence and all three men for everything they've taught me.

I'd also like to deeply appreciate the wisdom, love and example of my therapist, supervisor and trainers Rex Bradley, Jenner Roth and Terry Cooper at Spectrum. I have a huge debt to them and to all the gay men, lesbians and bisexuals I've been privileged to work with.

We would both like to thank:

- Don Clark and Celestial Arts for permission to quote from *The New Loving Someone Gay* (1987).

x Acknowledgements

- Anthony Hillin and the Central Council for Education and Training in Social Work (CCETSW) for permission to reproduce the two diagrams on internalized oppression in Chapter 3 which came from the document *Sexuality, Young People and Care* (Bremner and Hillin 1993).
- Fran Walsh for permission to use her 'Cycle of oppression' (1992), p. 47.
- Werner Ullah for allowing us to use the title which he inaugurated for a journal about lesbian and gay therapy issues for therapists connected to the Westminster Pastoral Foundation's training programmes.

CHARLES NEAL AND DOMINIC DAVIES

Introduction

The need for this book

It is only a few years since homosexuality has been declassified as a mental illness in the UK (*ICD* 1992), although it was declassified two decades ago in the USA. There are still many professionals 'treating' people for homosexuality and many more who, whilst they 'know' there is no 'treatment' available, believe that homosexuality is in some way abnormal or disordered. There is also now a large group of professionals who feel sure same sex sexuality is not pathological but who lack the information they need to contradict prejudicial learning from their culture and their own psychological or therapeutic training.

Whilst issues in transcultural and multiracial counselling have recently begun to be addressed, little, if anything, has been done around lesbian and gay issues in therapy. Rarely are sexual minorities covered in training programmes and yet increasing numbers of lesbian, gay and bisexual clients are presenting for therapy. Some argue that lesbians, gay men and bisexuals are overrepresented in the client population of some services (see Ratigan this volume); others have found the experience of living with a stigmatized identity has contributed to lower levels of psychological well-being than the general population (Coyle 1993). There is therefore a pressing need for therapists and other helping professionals to respond more appropriately and in order to do this effectively, they need training.

The most accessible form of training in gay affirmative therapy issues at the present is likely to be through reading. This is the first British book to cover these issues. This book is for those who wish to learn more. It is also for all who wish to ensure that their work values clients of all sexual orientations equally. We have not set out to persuade those whose value systems require them to believe homosexuality to be wrong to change their minds. It is unlikely they will read this book but in case they do, we ask them to consider how appropriate it is to be working with clients with whom they cannot offer the core ethic of *respect*.

The declassification of homosexuality in the United States has allowed gay affirmative models of therapy to develop. This work, initially inspired by peer counselling services and subsequently by qualified professionals, has led to much of the research that forms the basis of this book. Unfortunately, this is almost exclusively American and British therapists need to be aware that some of it may not translate directly to work in Britain. However, the contributors to this volume have all worked in the UK for a number of years and endeavoured to include information that *they* have found useful in their clinical practice; often they illustrate their points through clinical examples.

One of us began training as a therapist over a decade ago and was often the only person from a sexual minority on courses or workshops, personally experiencing a great deal of isolation and well meant 'curiosity' and at other times ignorance and homophobia. As this book was being finished, we continued to hear accounts of therapists in training asked, 'Why do you feel the need to proclaim your sexuality?' and 'Surely we're all non-judgmental and gay people are just the same as the rest of us, so why do we need training to work with them?' Few British training courses in counselling or psychotherapy cover working with lesbian, gay and bisexual people; some may explore attitudes to sexual minorities, but rarely will they look at clinical issues. When they do it is our experience that courses usually offer an hour or two, and at best a day's workshop. Gay people comprise around 10 per cent of the population. This book clearly demonstrates that we have psychological and emotional issues not faced by our heterosexual peers. The reader is invited to judge whether the training needs of therapists, counsellors and other health professionals are being adequately served by this level of specialist input.

Aims

We seek to provide an overview of why lesbian, gay and bisexual therapy is an area worthy of the attention of counsellors and therapists, as well as to discuss some common clinical issues. A model of gay affirmative therapy will be proposed which builds on some of the ideas and research developed in the past 20 years by practitioners. We attempt to make links between 'gay affirmative' and more explicitly humanistic or psychodynamic theoretical models. We also provide information on resources available to support therapists and clients as well as recommending further reading.

The book aims to do four things:

1 provide counsellors and therapists with knowledge about same sex sexuality and its social contexts and outline the history of psychological thinking about these;
2 distinguish affirmative and non-affirmative frameworks for therapeutic practice;
3 provide an understanding of some of the common clinical issues in working with lesbians, gay men and bisexual people;
4 help readers consider and work on their own feelings and attitudes to lesbians, gay men and bisexual people and offer guidelines for (re)training.

Limitations

Ethnic diversity

This book has been written by predominantly white therapists although we are of varied European ethnicity. The material we have used in this book comes from two sources: empirical research (usually from the United States), and our own clinical and personal experiences. American research into working with people from minority ethnic backgrounds tends to revolve around African-American or Hispanic identities which bear little relevance to British, or even European, black communities. We have endeavoured to reflect the experience of black people in our case studies and in research where relevant. At present there are few black lesbian, gay or bisexual therapists working in our communities and this loss to our profession is also a weakness with this book. We hope that this lack will encourage black lesbian, gay and bisexual therapists to write about their experiences. This is sorely needed.

Bisexuality: a new political and cultural identity

Research has shown that over time, most people are attracted sexually (at least intrapsychically) to both genders. Few people exhibit an exclusive sexual orientation. Yet the myth of dichotomous sexualities continues to be pushed by both the heterosexual and homosexual communities. This is distinctly unhelpful since it creates a false division into what is acceptable and is extremely inaccurate.

Many people who define themselves as heterosexual have sex with their own gender. Even more have sexual fantasies or dreams about doing so. Many lesbians and gay men have sex with the opposite sex, yet define themselves as lesbian or gay. This is not new information. We have known it for many hundreds of years, and yet continue to divide ourselves from one another, or internally from our own other sexual parts. It is becoming more common for us to talk about 'lesbian wives and mothers' and 'married gay men' than people being bisexual.

In this book we will continue to address those people who have same sex relations as lesbian or gay and request the reader to remember that the majority of us have a sexual orientation which is not fixed and will involve most of us at some stage thinking about, and possibly actually having, sexual relationships with both genders.

The areas covered by this book apply to those of us who would define ourselves as lesbian, gay or bisexual. Where we know of a specific difference for bisexuals we will endeavour to make mention of it. However, since most research into human sexuality has fallen into the trap of the dichotomous view of sexuality, then most attention has focused on lesbians and gay men, and unfortunately scant attention paid to bisexuality.

Over the past 10 years, in particular, there have been increasing numbers of men and women coming out as bisexual and carving out identities separate from, but often affiliated to, lesbian and gay identities. There has been a great deal of resistance to bisexuality, which is seen as threatening to many heterosexuals because of the homosexual component, and threatening to some lesbians and gay men because bisexuals are seen to be retaining the privileges and respectability of heterosexuals. This anti-bisexual sentiment has come to be known as '*biphobia*'; although not strictly accurate, it seems more accessible than 'anti-bisexualism'. Both homophobia and heterosexism militate against people coming out publicly as bisexual.

Bisexuals have often fought alongside lesbians and gay men for sexual equality, and have socialized in lesbian and gay environments where their homosexuality has been accepted. However, most have had to deny that part of them that is heterosexual in these situations, in the same way that many lesbians and gay men have had to deny their homosexuality in oppressive heterosexual settings. The emergence of a bisexual community with its own publications, politics, culture, conferences, support groups and meeting places means that bisexuals can find full acceptance and affirmation of their right to love both men and women.

HIV and AIDS issues

We decided not to include a chapter on HIV and AIDS issues separately for a number of reasons. This area of work and interest has generated a huge amount of literature itself and continues to do so. The different issues in HIV therapy warrant separate attention. The frequent conflation of HIV and AIDS issues with those arising from the experience of minority sexual identity has been damaging to both areas of focus. AIDS and HIV are not only important for lesbians, gay men and bisexuals, nor are they our only important issues; indeed, lesbians are less likely to be affected by them than heterosexual women or men, except in the key area of bereavement due to loss of gay male friends. Too often when same sex sexuality is raised in training or clinical discussion, the focus quickly becomes AIDS and HIV related.

A starting point

All of the areas covered by the chapters here merit considerably more research, discussion and literature. We know that many other topics of concern to gay men, lesbians and bisexual people have not been covered at all. This book seeks merely to start the debate on this side of the Atlantic. We look forward enthusiastically to many more books on these matters and to further reputable research. We welcome the widest possible dissemination of clinical experience. It is our hope that ethical practitioners in alliance with increasingly informed clients from sexual minorities will insist on changes in training, ethics, attitudes and legislation in order to guarantee equality of psychological care for all.

The structure and uses of the book

We recommend that Part I of the book be considered essential reading. Our aim here has been to address the meaning of sexual orientation and to explore the history of attitudes in psychology towards sexual minorities, as well as to offer an outline of more respectful, 'gay affirmative' models for therapeutic trainings and practices. We have particularly considered readers who do not themselves identify as lesbian, gay or bisexual, and their need for information about sexual minority lifestyles, cultures and psychological experiences.

Part II consists of chapters by different authors on specific issues affecting lesbian, gay and bisexual clients generally, such as making relationships work and family issues, as well as some conflicts or difficulties experienced by smaller numbers of clients, for example, partner abuse or problems with substance use.

The first part of this book is core reading, a background for chapters from Part II which are of particular interest. Appendices 1 and 2 add information on resources available to support clients and therapists and Appendix 3 recommends further reading on the topics discussed in each chapter. Finally there is an extensive references section which we hope will serve as a valuable resource for colleagues interested in further research.

What's in a name?

Gay and lesbian

A great many homosexual women and men now refer to themselves as 'lesbian' or 'gay'. This is an important statement of self-definition and a move away from medical pathology. Far fewer lesbians and gay men have attempted to counteract stigma and self-identify by using previously pejorative terms themselves, describing themselves as 'dykes' and 'queers', for example. It is important for therapists wishing to establish constructive working relationships to use the terms clients have adopted for themselves. We have generally used 'lesbian' and 'gay' unless writing historically and have often simply used 'clients', as the whole book is about lesbian, gay and bisexual clients specifically.

Therapists and counsellors

We use the term 'therapist' as a shorthand to describe psychotherapists and counsellors of any theoretical orientation. The term is also intended to embrace advice workers, health professionals, social workers and other helping practitioners whose interest in these matters includes them in our readership.

Defining terms

Most chapters begin by defining special terms used. This is to ensure that the reader develops a common understanding with the writer. It was our preference to develop mutual ground in this way, beginning with some key terms in the core first section and introducing others as the topic required it, rather than providing a glossary which we felt would possibly oversimplify and decontextualize.

Case examples

We use clinical examples to illustrate theoretical material. These are usually composites from a number of clients' stories (unless otherwise stated) and have been thoroughly disguised. There are a few exceptions (as where clients and therapists discuss working with heterosexual trainers and therapists in Chapter 3) and here explicit permission from the source has been granted. We hope all examples serve as helpful illustrations of the points being made and all contributors have made every effort not to describe clients as if they were intrinsically different from ourselves in their issues, struggles and experiences.

The future

We earnestly hope this book contributes to your own future thinking and practice and that you will in turn participate in challenging oppression. There is increasing activity and interest amongst client groups, sexual minority communities and professionals of all theoretical and sexual orientations in the issues raised here. We are ourselves involved in many ways (see Notes on Contributors) and would be interested to hear from readers about future developments in Britain and other European countries particularly aimed at ending the stigmatization and abuse of those from sexual minority groups.

PART I

Fundamental issues

| 1 | DOMINIC DAVIES WITH
CHARLES NEAL

An historical overview of homosexuality and therapy

This chapter examines the relationship of therapy to homosexuality. We propose to explore some of the difficulties in conducting research into homosexuality, and look at how some therapists have responded to troubled lesbian, gay and bisexual clients.

Defining sexuality

In discussing homosexuality, it is helpful for therapists to have an understanding of the difference between *homosexual behaviour* (having sex with someone of the same sex) and *homosexual identity* (seeing oneself as homosexual). The term homosexuality will, however, be used to include those who self-define as homosexual as well as those whose sexual behaviour may include same sex relationships, but whose current sexual identity is not homo-, or bisexual. We are doing this in the interests of simplicity and because, for some of those whose behaviour includes same sex sexual activity, their identity may later change to something which more fully reflects their practice (i.e. they haven't 'come out' yet).

The significance of separating behaviour from identity becomes apparent when we try to examine the incidence of homosexuality. The majority of the population do not describe their sexuality in a way which is congruent with their behaviour and fantasies. The foremost work on the incidence of homosexuality was conducted by Alfred Kinsey and colleagues (1947, 1953). Kinsey reported that 37 per cent of males and 13 per cent of females had, as adults, engaged in sexual contact to orgasm with a member of the same sex. In the same samples, only 4 per cent of males and between 0.3 and

3.0 per cent of females reported themselves to be *exclusively* homosexual. It should be remembered that this data reflects a particular sample of 20,000 people in post-war America, but other surveys have reported similar levels (4–6 per cent) of exclusive homosexuality (Gebhard 1972; Meyer 1985). Gonsiorek and Weinrich (1991) cite a cross-cultural study (Sell *et al.* 1990) of same sex behaviour of men from France, the United Kingdom and the United States in which 11.6 per cent, 7.8 per cent and 11.6 per cent of subjects respectively reported same sex sexual behaviour from the age of 15. Furthermore, 10.8 per cent, 4.7 per cent and 6.3 per cent respectively reported same sex sexual behaviour within the previous five years. They state:

> This... is a powerful study, as it randomly surveyed large numbers of subjects (more than 5,700 roughly evenly divided among the three countries) and used well-trained field staff personally interviewing subjects. It can therefore stand as reasonably sound current national prevalence data.
>
> (Gonsiorek and Weinrich 1991: 4)

We can see, therefore, that some people are likely, due to social pressures, to underreport their same sex behaviour, but that approximately 7–12 per cent of the population 'admit' to having sex with someone of the same sex more than once. Kinsey (1947) found similar numbers of exclusive heterosexuals to his exclusive homosexual subjects, thereby demonstrating a much higher proportion of people than expected who were bisexual in behaviour and fantasy, if not in identity.

Bisexuality

There has been a spurious assumption on the part of many researchers and practitioners that people are either homo- or heterosexual. We know from the above prevalence studies that this is not the case, but for a variety of reasons these divisions continue. Since much of the research into homosexuality has focused on either self-identity *or* behaviour, people who have sexual relationships with both sexes may have been counted within the research into homosexuality. At other times people who have both same and opposite sex relationships may have been excluded from the data. This has served to blur what we know about lesbians and gay men, as well as obscuring accurate research into bisexuality. We believe it is important to conduct research into bisexual psychology to see how it compares with lesbian and gay psychologies. In the absence of such evidence, we are assuming that the psychology of bisexuals is not very different to that of lesbians and gay men.

Gay 'identity'

Anthropologists have demonstrated (e.g. Weinrich and Williams 1991) that homosexual behaviour occurs in all cultures throughout the world. In some it is approved of, even encouraged. Homosexuality has different cultural meanings and is understood in different ways throughout the world.

In the western world, we have developed the concept of a 'gay identity', a set of cultural beliefs, values and support networks, institutions, artefacts and languages which contribute towards subcultures, of which modern lesbians or gay men can identify themselves as members (see Weeks 1985 for more on this). Because of the way homosexuality is seen in other cultures, we may not find a similar 'gay identity'. However, as Weinrich and Williams (1991: 45), point out:

> the more a culture is studied, the more different patterns of homosexuality or homosexual behaviour turn up in it, and the more this range of behaviour seems similar to the range (if not the proportions) observed in other cultures, including Western culture.

It has clearly been documented that homosexuality is a universally occurring phenomenon, but is it 'natural'? One objection to homosexuality is that it is unnatural. Some moral theologians attempt to use poor biology to show that this is so. Kirsch and Weinrich (1991) demonstrate from a sociobiological perspective that homosexuality is natural, and go on to suggest that it may even be part of an evolutionary purpose. They explore the possible biological and genetic basis for homosexuality where the goal of evolutionary success is reproductive fitness, and ask how, if homosexuals reproduce less, does homosexuality survive?

> By definition, natural selection ought to eliminate any gene predisposing toward or even permitting the expression of homosexual behaviour extensive enough to interfere with or reduce reproduction.
> (Kirsch and Weinrich 1991: 22)

The research

There has been a great deal of research into (male) homosexuality. This has involved a variety of scientists including biologists, psychologists, anthropologists, and sociologists and readers may well be familiar with many of the alleged 'causes' derived from this activity. The theories about the causes of homosexuality can be loosely divided into biological (nature) and environmental (nurture) ones:

Nature: too much or too little sex hormone (oestrogen, testosterone, androgen); an extra gene; a smaller or larger hypothalamus; maternal stress during pregnancy; different sizes of various sections of the brain.

Nurture: overprotective, overdemanding and close binding mothers; absent or distant fathers; a fear of, or a negative experience with, the other sex; single-sex schools; a positive first sexual experience with the same sex; seduction by an older homosexual; sexual abuse; being reared in a household with too many siblings of the other sex; women teachers; loud disco music and eating the meat of uncircumcised pigs!

We do not propose to cite the above researchers, since much of this research is faulty, and therefore inconsequential and would overload the references index. Those interested in some of the major theories around the development of homosexuality would do well to study Ruse (1988) for a critical overview.

Behind much of the research into homosexuality is the search for aetiology (pathology), which presupposes that if one can find the cause, one can then find a 'cure'. This 'medical model', whilst somewhat outdated now, has previously attracted a great deal of attention. The belief that there is something abnormal about a homosexual orientation which needs correcting or treating is unfortunately still common to many people. Various treatments have been used to attempt to cure or correct a homosexual orientation, including electric shock treatment, brain surgery, castration, hormone injections and other biochemical therapies, and a variety of psychotherapies, most notably long term psychoanalysis. Surprisingly perhaps, none of these 'treatments' has been proven to effect a long term conversion or reorientation to heterosexuality, and so far the search for a single causal factor has been fruitless. However, the search still goes on. Current research is concentrating on the biological basis of homosexuality, and work is being conducted in the fields of genetics and endocrinology, particularly around prenatal hormones.

Flaws in methodology

Some of the difficulties lie in how the questions are asked and by whom. One of the leading pieces of psychoanalytic work on male homosexuality for example was by Beiber and colleagues (1962) who used questionnaires which were completed not by the subjects themselves but by their analysts based on what their patients had told them. It will be obvious to most therapists that we only see the part of our clients' lives that they want us to see, and know what they have chosen to tell us.

Other research has used telephone surveys, or face to face interviews. Bearing in mind the continuing guilt, stigma and embarrassment associated with homosexuality, it is likely that underreporting will be common using these methods. Concern for confidentiality, rapport between interviewer and subject and the subjective impressions the subject has of the interviewer all have to be borne in mind. A further methodological obstacle with asking people explicit questions about their sexual behaviour is around anonymity. Gonsiorek and Weinrich (1991: 4) comment:

> A major problem facing such studies is the risk involved in self-disclosure, especially where the studies fail to ensure complete anonymity. It is possible, indeed quite likely, that these recurrent 2–6 per cent figures [of homosexual identity] represent an absolute minimum and that they represent homosexual individuals who are relatively open and who live in tolerant, or cosmopolitan communities.

Another common method of evaluating data is the use of self-completed questionnaires. It may be useful to consider the motivations of people willing to volunteer to participate in sex research and self-administering questionnaires, since perhaps they are a biased sample too. Much of the early research into causes of homosexuality comes from research with unhappy and troubled people who presented for help with their identity, and access to representative samples of 'non-patient' groups of lesbians, gays and bisexuals is extremely difficult: one begins to form an impression of some of the methodological constraints.

To be able to rely on any research into incidence of homosexuality one needs to have a number of research methods, perhaps including some corroborative and objective tests. One research instrument developed by Freund (1974) that can help provide objective evidence of homosexual interest is the *plethysmograph*, which is a device that fits over the penis and measures changes in blood volume. A similar device has been developed to measure female genital blood flow. Sexual orientation can be observed by showing the subject photographs of naked people of various ages and appearances and of both sexes. The plethysmograph, unsurprisingly, only works with willing participants. It is therefore impractical to use it on the general population. It does have some use to ascertain the incidence of homosexuality amongst a group of volunteer subjects, but again one would have to wonder about the motivation of the volunteers. Were they sexually less inhibited anyway, and could higher indices of homosexuality amongst such groups be due to their lowered inhibitions?

One key question for the therapist reading any research into 'causes' or 'cures' is: 'How was the sample obtained?' The second question to ask is: 'Why is this research being carried out, and what value does it have?' Although value is obviously a subjective concept, it might be useful to consider whose needs are being served.

Research into lesbianism has been much more recent, if no more welcome: see Val Young's introduction to Chapter 9. It is interesting to note that no research has been officially carried out into the 'causes' of heterosexuality, or how heterosexuals might be helped to overcome their 'obsession' with only responding to the other sex! An interesting questionnaire for heterosexual readers to consider is at the end of the book (Appendix 1). The questionnaire has been taken from some suggested exercises for heterosexism awareness workshops, and through use of irony turns questions often asked of lesbians and gay men into questions for heterosexuals on their sexuality.

The researchers: the ethics of 'causes' and 'cures'

Motivation of researchers

It may be helpful to consider what motivates someone to spend a great deal of time, effort and money in research. Obviously some therapists began working with unhappy homosexuals because they wanted to help their clients. They naïvely located the clients' difficulties as their homosexuality, rather than helping the client deal with society's homophobia. The motivation behind some of the people currently researching into the causes of homosexuality, however, is clearly morally biased and sinister. The aim for the eradication of homosexuality is present in Gunter Dörner's work in Germany where he was investigating the use of the drug Lisuride to 'cure' homosexuality in rats:

> It was concluded from these data that ... it might become possible in the future – at least in some cases – to correct abnormal sex hormone levels during brain differentiation in order to *prevent the development of homosexuality*. However, this should be done, if at all, only if it is urgently desired by the pregnant mother.
> (Dörner 1983, as quoted in Silverstein 1991: 108, emphasis added)

Others have breached their professional association's code of ethics in their pursuit for causes of homosexuality and misrepresentation of scientific fact. This has led in at least one case (Paul Cameron of Nebraska) to dismissal from membership of the American Psychological Association (Herek 1991: 80). However, this has clearly not deterred Cameron who continues to publish research which misrepresents homosexuality (Cameron 1985; Cameron *et al.* 1986).

When New York professor of psychiatry, Charles Socarides, was invited to Britain in 1995 by several training establishments to discuss homosexuality as a 'sickness' and describe how he 'cures' his gay patients, many in and outside the field of psychology were horrified to discover these views being given serious attention by, for example, the main analytic association within the National Health Service. Our third chapter deals in greater detail with homophobia.

Krajeski (1986: 22) puts the situation quite clearly for many people:

An historical overview of homosexuality and therapy 17

Although it may be to the advantage of gay people to be viewed as healthy rather than as mentally disturbed, such a view may damage the credibility of experts who have built a reputation on understanding homosexuality as a mental disorder. As gay men and women stand to gain in self-respect and credibility, others stand to lose these same qualities.

More recently there has been research from gay scientists. Gay geneticist Simon Le Vay (1993) believes he has found a part of gay men's brains which is different to heterosexual men's brains. Whether or not he is correct, his motivation seems to be to try to prove that homosexuality is innate and therefore beyond our control, in the way that eye colour is beyond our control. Legislation could then prevent discrimination against lesbians and gay men for something which is inherent, and about which they have no choice.

This argument is somewhat flawed. First, many would argue that race and sex equality legislation has actually done very little to prevent discrimination against people of colour or women (for example, women are still on average paid less than men; black people are still more likely to receive custodial sentences than white offenders). Second, as discussed earlier (Kinsey *et al.* 1947), the majority of people who have same sex sexual relationships have also had sex with the other gender. Many people shift in their sexual orientation over time and so Le Vay is trying to find a 'cause' of homosexuality for that proportion of lesbians and gay men (4–6 per cent) who remain *exclusively* homosexual. Third, Le Vay's research was only conducted on brains of men; it has no relevance to the cause of lesbianism and would, presumably, have marginal relevance to bisexuality.

The ethics of treatment

Some therapists have attempted to 'cure' lesbians, gays and bisexuals of their homosexuality, sometimes known as 'conversion'. There is a history of 'treatments' that are akin to methods of torture which interested readers can follow up for themselves through the excellent critical reviews of the research provided by Gonsiorek (1981), Blair (1982), Davison (1991), Haldeman (1991), and Silverstein (1991). Notions of 'cure' and 'treatment' derive, of course, from quasi-medical models of homosexuality as a 'sickness' or 'disease'. Over 100 years' struggle to find a scientific basis for this view having failed, it is remarkable how durable these prejudices are within professions claiming a primary interest in human health and well-being. For most of the twentieth century 'medical' models have, perhaps, seemed preferable to models of good and evil, which they largely replaced.

Even in the past two decades the 'cures' have included neurosurgery, peripheral hormone injections, psychoanalysis, aversion therapy using electric shocks and nausea inducing drugs, social learning and heterosexual assertiveness training, religious exorcism and prayer. Needless to say, none of these methods have proved effective in the 'conversion' of exclusive homosexuals into heterosexuals. A number of ethical issues arise from them. Krajeski (1986: 21), pertinently asks, 'Is it acceptable to treat a condition which is not an illness, but which society condemns?' and Begelman (1975), in a critique of behaviour therapy which could apply to any therapeutic intervention aimed at 'conversion', states:

> [The efforts of behaviour therapists to re-orient homosexuals to heterosexuality] *by their very existence constitute a significant causal element in reinforcing the social doctrine that homosexuality is bad.* Indeed, the point of the activist protest is that behaviour therapists contribute significantly to preventing the exercise of any *real* option in decision making about sexual identity, by further strengthening the prejudices that homosexuality is a 'problem behaviour', since treatment may be offered for it. As a consequence of this therapeutic stance, as well as a wider system of social and attitudinal pressures, homosexuals tend to seek treatment *for being homosexuals.*
> (Begelman 1975: 180 quoted by Haldeman 1991: 141–2)

Davison (1978), a behaviourist who is also concerned about ethics, argues that even the availability of change of orientation programmes causes hurt and damage to individuals both in and outside of therapy.

Christian 'conversion'

Most respectable therapists would refuse to collude with a client's wish for 'cure', and instead work with them on the self-loathing and help them come to terms, and cope more effectively, with societal homophobia. A major threat to this somewhat idealistic view lies in religious counselling programmes aimed at spiritual salvation and known in many quarters as the 'ex-gay movement'. These groups actively recruit, through media campaigns and relationships with Christian psychiatrists and therapists, more vulnerable lesbians, gays and bisexuals for 'healing and cure' of their sexuality. Evidence of vulnerability was provided by Weinberg and Williams (1974), who found that gay men for whom religion was very important were likely to view homosexuality as sinful, have lower self-concepts, show higher levels of depression and to feel a greater sense of apprehension about being 'found out' and how others might react to them. Chapter 13 of this book discusses this issue further.

There is no reliable research evidence that religious programmes can 'cure' homosexuality; there is plenty of evidence that the leaders of these programmes have a history of dubious sexual ethics and are responsible for severe psychological damage to people seeking their help. (Blair 1982 documents this well and Haldeman 1991 provides further evidence.) What is more, these 'treatments' are unethical:

> Psychological ethics mandate that mental health professionals subscribe to methods that support human dignity and are effective in their stated purpose. Conversion therapy qualifies as neither. It reinforces the social stigma associated with homosexuality, and there is no evidence from any of the studies reviewed here to suggest that sexual orientation can be changed.
> (Haldeman 1991: 159)

Most Christians, of course, clergy and lay, men and women, homosexual and heterosexual, would wish to be totally dissociated from these anti-gay sentiments and the 'treatment' programmes that stem from them.

Therapy's relationship to homosexuality

In 1935 Freud replied to a letter from an American mother who had sought his help for her homosexual son:

> Homosexuality is assuredly no advantage, but it is nothing to be ashamed of, no vice, no degradation, it cannot be classified as an illness ... Many highly respectable individuals of ancient and modern times have been homosexuals, several of the greatest men among them (Plato, Michelangelo, Leonardo da Vinci, etc.). It is a great injustice to persecute homosexuality as a crime, and a cruelty too.
> (Freud 1947: 786–7)

This seems a fairly enlightened reply from the originator of an approach which has sometimes been responsible for atrocities in the name of therapy. We quote it to draw the reader's attention to an early and sympathetic response from the founder of psychotherapy. Freud clearly had much to say about homosexuality, and a critique of his theories can be found in Ruse (1988). However, for his time, Freud was saying that the aim of therapy with homosexuals was to facilitate self-acceptance. This aim would be shared by contemporary gay affirmative therapists.

There have been a lot of patients on the couch since Freud's reply to the American mother, and homosexuality was still classified as a mental disorder by the World Health Organization under the International Classification of Diseases (ICD) until the 10th edition in 1992. This is the system of classification of mental illness that applies to British psychiatrists and psychologists. In the United States, the equivalent system of the American Psychiatric Association (APA) is known as the Diagnostic Statistical Manual (DSM) (American Psychiatric Association 1980). Homosexuality *per se* was declassified by the APA as a mental disorder in 1973, only to be replaced in 1980 by a new category of *ego-dystonic homosexuality*. This new and confusing classification was dropped in the revision of DSM III published in 1987, being replaced by *sexual disorder not otherwise specified* defined by 'persistent and marked distress about one's sexual orientation'. It is difficult to imagine how many people who are not in fact homosexual or bisexual would be classified this way.

Psychoanalysis begins with a contradiction about human sexuality and this has yet to be resolved. Freud's 'Three Essays on the Theory of Sexuality' (1905) separated sexual practices from gender, thus founding a radical and invaluable new way of talking and thinking about these matters. However, he had to acknowledge his own inability to enter this new discourse completely and to forego holding on to notions of masculinity and femininity as if they were biological categories (Freud 1913). Freud recognized that Oedipal theory, central to his project, depended on the maintenance of what Sinfield (1994) calls 'the cross-sex grid' – that is, continuing bipolar explanations of genders and sexualities as 'opposite' to one another. Readers interested in the historical construction of sexualities will find fascinating material in Weeks (1985: Parts II and III) and Dollimore (1991: 170–5, 205–12, 253–60) as well as Sinfield (1994: Chapter 7).

These two strands in the therapeutic traditions – one open to diversity of sexual experience and expression and the other conserving older frameworks for the classification and systemizing of gender and sexuality – absorb us still. The 'conservative' one has its origins in nineteenth-century concerns with social power over what is deemed 'healthy' and the early sexologist's pseudoscientific descriptions of 'perversions'; this chapter notes some current repercussions of this inheritance.

Guy Hocquenghem argues that psychoanalysis now constitutes 'the most amazing system of guilt inducement ever invented' and 'a system of oppression of one sexual mode, the heterosexual family mode, over all possible other modes' (Hocquenghem 1978: 59, 124). There is increasing dissatisfaction in and outside the fields of theory and therapy, with dialogues modelled on Victorian analytic dominance (see, for example, Masson 1984 and Kitzinger and Perkins 1993). There has been clear empirical evidence that homosexuality is not pathological, and that lesbians and gay men have the mental health equivalent to heterosexuals since Evelyn Hooker's rigorous study in 1957. Further and more varied research was conducted over the subsequent two decades and has been reviewed by Gonsiorek (1977), Hart *et al.* (1978) and Reiss (1980); the interested reader is invited to pursue this independently.

The American psychoanalyst Richard Isay (1989) notes that the antihomosexual bias had its roots nourished in the American psychoanalytic tradition. He believes this occurred because during World War II a number of analysts occupied senior positions in military psychiatry. The military feared that sexual attraction within and between the ranks would interfere with discipline, an anxiety which still besets the American and British armed forces! After the war these analysts became influential in psychiatry, heading departments in hospitals, chairing professional committees and so on.

> After the war they consolidated the gains they had made in achieving a significant degree of respectability for the new science of psychoanalysis by further strengthening its ties to psychiatry, medicine and the disease model.
>
> (Isay 1989: 6)

Importantly too, a large number of European analysts fleeing Nazi persecution went to the United States. These refugees needed to be accepted and to feel secure in their new country. Many, who in Europe were outspoken and radical free thinkers, because of the Cold War, McCarthyism and the need to become assimilated now allied themselves with organized American psychoanalysis. The medical model held there committed them to orthodoxy and social conformity. Isay (1989: 6) cites Clarence Oberndorf, an ex-president of the American Psychoanalytic Association, as saying:

> Psychoanalysis had finally become legitimate and respectable, perhaps paying the price in becoming sluggish and smug, hence attractive to an increasing number of minds which found security in conformity.

During the same period Isay (1989: 7) notes that:

> when there were purges of homosexuals from government, there was also consolidation within psychoanalysis of the theory of the pathological adaptation of homosexuals, and the exclusion of homosexuals from analytic institutes became customary.

This American experience was echoed in Europe. The Nazis, for example, had conducted numerous experiments on gay men incarcerated in concentration camps. *The Hidden Holocaust* (Grau 1995) details the horrifying history of this. It arose from 100 years of supposedly scientific experimentation, informed by and reinforcing prevailing sexological orthodoxy.

The more radical tradition, the one Freud wished to be able to embrace more fully himself, 'prides itself on its capacity to question, to pursue the idea behind the idea, to be curious rather than censorious, to acknowledge the transgressive and socially inconvenient... is in principle a place of discovery' (Orbach 1995: 8) and is also alive and, in some places, well.

The separation of human sexuality from gender (Freud 1905) provides the background for gender and sexuality studies today and for models of affirmative therapy such as those that are the subject of this book (see Chapter 3 especially). Isay (1989) goes quite some way to construct a reworking of Freudian theory, while Sinfield (1994) argues that a new framework altogether is needed to challenge the dominance of Victorian normative discourses. Lesbian, gay and bisexual clients will continue meanwhile to feel apprehensive and suspicious about psychology, analysis, therapy and related research. Until certain conditions are seen to have changed considerably, they will not expect to find their integrity validated.

One particularly significant area where change is urgently needed is in the training of therapists. It is still the situation today that gay men and lesbians are usually excluded from being able to train as psychoanalysts in the US and Britain, due to their 'unresolved and unanalysable neuroses'. Ellis (1994) found in her research into psychoanalytically oriented training establishments in Britain that, in spite of reluctance to admit to refusing admission to a programme because someone was lesbian or gay, she had evidence of heterosexist bias, beliefs that homosexuality equated with psychopathology, and the fact that an 'out' lesbian or gay man would be regarded as 'too political' and therefore 'inappropriate' for training. The interested reader may well want to follow up her research, and that of O'Connor and Ryan (1993) who have re-examined the major psychoanalytic theories around homosexuality. Chapter 2 sets out guidelines for the (re)training of all therapists; this is necessary if clients of all sexualities are to be accorded equal respect.

Conclusions

- Whilst some people define themselves as lesbian, gay or bisexual, others, in spite of having same sex sexual experiences, do not.
- It is extremely difficult to conduct reliable research into the incidence of homosexuality (both behaviour and identity), but our best 'guesstimates' seem to show that about 10 per cent of the population are homosexual and a larger number will have some experience of same sex sexual relationships.
- Homosexuality has been researched for over a century by modern science and there still is no dependable research to inform us why some people are homosexual and others are not.
- Homosexuals appear to have similar levels of mental health as heterosexuals, and years of 'treatment' have brought years of suffering.
- Psychology and psychoanalytic theory have often contributed towards reinforcing prejudice and polarizing sexualities in the past with some cruel and unethical results.
- People of all sexualities have the right to equal respect, value and integrity.
- There is an urgent need for training in therapy to end heterosexist discrimination.

- The role of the modern therapist is the same as Freud described it in his letter in 1935: to help the person make the most of their life; to explore, affirm and integrate their sexuality. How we can work in this self-affirming way with homosexual and bisexual clients (gay affirmative therapy) is the subject of this book.

2 | DOMINIC DAVIES

Towards a model of gay affirmative therapy

This chapter seeks to present a model for working with clients who identify as lesbian, gay or bisexual which does not pathologize or discriminate against such clients. The aim is to present therapists, regardless of theoretical orientation, with a set of guidelines and tenets for effective and respectful therapeutic work which will enable them to create positive relationships with these clients as with others, and to propose these guidelines be used as a basis for retraining therapists whose only training to date has reinforced dominant cultural stereotyping. When one takes account of homophobia and heterosexism evident in some psychological theory, practice and research (as discussed in other chapters), the significance of the development of a different model will be clear.

Gay affirmative therapy

The purpose of these tenets and guidelines is to augment the deficits and heterosexist assumptions of the major theoretical therapy models. These have led, as we have seen earlier, to unethical, invasive and abusive practices at times and to the exclusion of lesbian, gay and bisexual people from training. Heterosexism is the belief that heterosexuality is superior to, or more natural or healthy than, other sexualities. This is discussed in detail in Chapter 3 on homophobia and heterosexism. I will assert that it is not enough simply to offer Rogers's (1951) *core conditions,* nor is it sufficient to have a sound understanding of psychodynamic or cognitive behavioural principles. This new 'model', which has been influenced by a number of therapists, largely in the United States, is one that deviates from some of the fundamental practices of the major schools, and therefore requires a name of its own.

Krajeski (1986: 16) points out the difficulty of finding a name 'which describes accurately a type of therapy which values both homosexuality and heterosexuality equally as natural or normal attributes'. The name with most common usage is *gay affirmative*. The gay affirmative therapist affirms a lesbian, gay or bisexual identity as an equally positive human experience and expression to heterosexual identity.

Maylon (1982: 69) describes gay affirmative therapy thus:

> Gay affirmative psychotherapy is not an independent system of psychotherapy. Rather it represents a special range of psychological knowledge which challenges the traditional view that homosexual desire and fixed homosexual orientations are pathological. Gay affirmative therapy uses traditional psychotherapeutic methods but proceeds from a non-traditional perspective. This approach regards homophobia, as opposed to homosexuality, as a major pathological variable in the development of certain symptomatic conditions among gay men.

Whilst I would agree that gay affirmative therapy is not an independent system, I suggest that there are some adjustments necessary to some of the more traditional schools of counselling and psychotherapy. Buhrke (1989) points out the heterosexist bias inherent in many traditional counselling theories and theories of personality development (e.g. Freud's genital stages and Erikson's Eight Ages of Man). Both the American psychoanalyst Richard Isay (1989) and the humanistic psychotherapist Don Clark (1987) state that therapeutic neutrality is both impossible (since we have all been exposed to society's negative messages about homosexuality) and oppressive. Isay believes that respect is central to the work with his gay clients, based on the belief that homosexuality is a normal and natural variation of human sexuality:

> I am emphasizing here the importance of the undeviatingly uncritical, accepting attitude in which the therapist's thoughtfulness, caring and regard for the patient are essential.
>
> (1989: 122)

I want to propose a model of gay affirmative therapy that can span the psychodynamic and humanistic schools. The skills and understandings of existing theoretical schools can be incorporated, augmenting them where necessary with gay affirmative concepts and current thinking on human sexuality.

The core condition of respect

Respect for the client's sexual orientation

This means that the therapist accepts that a homosexual or bisexual orientation is just as healthy as a heterosexual one; that homosexuality and bisexuality are natural variations on a continuum of human sexuality, and not pathological. Therapists need to think through their attitudes to sexuality *per se* and to reconsider archaic or naïve views of binary sexuality.

Respect for personal integrity

The therapist should strive towards a peer relationship with lesbian, gay and bisexual clients. Society has treated them in a pejorative way. It is helpful, therefore, for the therapist to seek to create a relationship which is collaborative, and become a companion in the client's journey, rather than the tour guide. This is based on the belief that the client knows what is best for them, or at least, if *they* do not know, the therapist certainly doesn't know.

> Help can be offered but not forced. Gay people have had too much damage done by would-be helpers who forced us to move in ways that we sensed were wrong or foreign to our nature. We will be rightly suspicious of help offered until we can sense its personal validity. You would do well to describe in advance what sort of help you intend to offer (in detail) and why. The lesbian/gay person will not truly accept help until a bond of trust has developed.
> (Clark 1987: 221)

This has implications for models of therapy which are based on the power and expertise of the therapist. For some practitioners of expert centred models, the therapist's power is central to the creation of a transference. It will be important for such therapists to consider the implications of this power in the light of the relative powerlessness and low self-esteem that many lesbian and gay clients experience. One very important aspect of respecting the client's integrity is that the therapist does not inform on the client by telling others – especially family.

> We gay people are keenly aware of how this information can be used against us and must choose for ourselves who and when to tell. Divulging information about gay identity is an absolute violation of trust as well as an ethical violation of confidentiality.
> (Clark 1987: 222)

This is also an important rule for social workers and teachers who may have contact with other members of the family.

The American therapist Marny Hall (1985) in her book *The Lavender Couch* suggests that lesbian, gay and bisexual people interview the potential therapist about the therapist's attitudes to, and training in, working with lesbian, gay and bisexual clients. This seems a sensible suggestion, since the client will be spending time, energy and not least money, on the work.

Appendix 1 includes a reproduction of the leaflet produced by the Association for Lesbian, Gay and Bisexual Psychologies on finding a gay affirmative therapist. Therapists can demonstrate their willingness to work alongside clients by answering such questions honestly and openly. The British Association for Counselling (BAC 1992) Code of Ethics and Practice states:

> B.2.2.8 Any publicity material and all written and oral information should reflect accurately the nature of the service on offer, and the training, qualifications and relevant experience of the counsellor.

Therapists who have been trained not to answer the client's questions, but rather to seek to understand what is behind the question and to remain what some psychodynamic practitioners have described as 'a blank screen', may find this difficult.

Respect for lifestyle and culture

Clients are entitled to respect for their culture and lifestyle. If a therapist feels unable to offer lesbian, gay and bisexual clients respect, then it is unethical for such therapists to work with them.

> It is an indication of the competence of counsellors when they recognise their inability to counsel a client or clients and make appropriate referrals.
> (BAC 1992: B.2.2.19)

It is important to examine one's ideas about values, morals and lifestyles when working with clients who are culturally different. It is probable that most lesbian, gay and bisexual clients are unlikely to share the lifestyle of their therapist, especially when she or he is heterosexual. There are a wide variety of lifestyles enjoyed by lesbians, gay men and bisexuals. Some live in relationships almost identical to heterosexual married couples, or very different (Chapter 6); others may live alone and have a variety of sexual partners, or none (Chapter 5).

It is important that therapists make every effort to learn for themselves about the diversity of lifestyles and cultures that exist within the lesbian, gay and bisexual communities and this is a major function of this book. It is inappropriate for a therapist to expect the client to 'teach' them about their lesbian, gay and bisexual lifestyle in general terms. The client is coming for therapy and, more often than not, paying for the service. It is unethical to expect them to provide the therapist with free consultancy on lesbian, gay and bisexual lifestyles and culture, unless they negotiate a reduction in their fee to reflect this!

Since therapy is about discovering and developing who one really is, some clients will be using therapy to try out different lifestyles. It is important that therapists respect their right to do this and to live their life their way.

We know being respected by someone else can be immensely freeing. Clients may feel as if they have permission to try out new ways of relating to themselves and others and different ways of living their lives, knowing that if these ways don't work out, they will not have lost face with their therapist.

Respectful attitudes and beliefs

Therapists have a duty to explore their own values for attitudes which may cause them difficulties *prior* to working with lesbian, gay and bisexual clients. They can then work on any prejudice in therapy or supervision or sensitively refer the client to another therapist. There should be no shame in deciding (for whatever reason) not to work with someone. In fact Woodman and Lenna (1980: 14) state:

> Gay clients have no desire to be confronted by therapists who warmly offer to help them make the best of a poor situation. In fact, such an attitude is one of the subtler forms of homophobia. Therapists who are unable to accept homosexuality as a positive and potentially creative way of being should recognize this fact and not treat gays, because their fear, anxiety, and ambivalence will inevitably be conveyed to their clients.

It is unrealistic for therapists to expect that they should be able to work with every client on any issue. It is a sign of professional integrity to be aware of one's prejudices and personal value systems and to refer a client elsewhere if it is anticipated that there may be conflicts. It is an indicator of professional incompetence to take on a client, where the therapist has (undeclared) prejudices or values which will clash with the client's value system and where respect for the client cannot be maintained. Some examples of beliefs that will make it impossible for a therapist to work respectfully with a lesbian, gay or bisexual client are:

- beliefs that homosexuality is against God's wishes, or sinful;
- beliefs that homosexuality is sick, unnatural or perverted;
- beliefs that homosexuality is a sad or inferior experience to heterosexuality;
- beliefs that monogamy is the only healthy way to conduct a sexual relationship;

- beliefs that homosexual relationships can only be shallow, or short lived, or sexual;
- beliefs that lesbian, gay and bisexual people are more likely to sexually abuse young people, or to 'pervert' their emergent sexualities in some way;
- beliefs that homosexual parenting or family lives are not real or of equal value with heterosexual equivalents.
- beliefs that bisexuals could decide to be homosexual or heterosexual instead.

If the therapist holds any of these beliefs then they should refrain from working with lesbian, gay and bisexual clients. If these notions are a valued part of the therapist's belief system they should refer these clients to someone who does not hold the same beliefs. It is the therapist's responsibility to find colleagues who do not feel as they do. If, however, the beliefs are left over from early socialization, then they should explore them in supervision, therapy, lesbian, gay and bisexual sensitivity training or through private study before, and independently of, working with these client groups.

Training and retraining

Working on the premise that lesbians and gay men are different but equal to heterosexuals and develop identities within cultures and subcultures of their own, just as people from minority ethnic communities do, then it is important that therapists are *trained* to work with them. Therapists need to be aware of their own homophobia and of the components of a lesbian or gay identity. Cayleff (1986), in discussing the ethical issues involved in counselling the culturally different (in which she includes lesbians, gay men and bisexuals), questions how therapists graduating from training programmes which do not require courses in working with the culturally different may ethically work with these populations.

Since 'education is a socialization process that imparts the values of the dominant culture' (Iasenza 1989: 73), the majority of counselling and therapy training programmes, through both course work and practice, continue to explore individual development, sex, gender, coupling, family and relationship issues solely within a heterosexual context.

Don Clark and his colleague Betty Berzon created a series of therapeutic guidelines for retraining to work with lesbian and gay clients (Clark 1987). Where there is conflict between an existing therapeutic model and the gay affirmative guideline when working with a lesbian, gay or bisexual client, the gay affirmative guideline should take precedence.

The purpose of retraining is twofold: (a) to explore one's own attitudes to homosexuality from a personal and professional perspective, and (b) to gain sufficient information regarding lesbian, gay and bisexual lifestyles and a sound understanding of homophobia and heterosexism.

It is presumptuous to assume that counselors who have been taught about valuable concepts like unconditional positive regard are able to apply them with gay–lesbian clients if they are not aware of their own heterosexual or homophobia biases.

(Iasenza 1989: 74)

Guidelines for gay affirmative practice

What follows is a discussion of the 'Twelve Guidelines for Retraining' and the 'Ground Rules for Helping' proposed by Clark (1987).

1 *'It is essential that you have developed a comfortable and appreciative orientation to your own homosexual feelings before you can work successfully with gay clients.'* It is not enough merely to be prepared to acknowledge one's homosexual feelings to oneself and others. We should be willing to honour these alongside general feelings of attraction for people of our own gender. We must be clear about our reasons for choosing seldom or never to act on them. Clark (1987: 233) maintains we all have homosexual feelings and:

> the professional who says he or she has no homosexual feelings [is] about as well off as the psychotherapist who says he or she never dreams. It indicates you are out of touch with your inner emotions and would do well to consider another profession.

This recommendation is not intended simply to be controversial. Therapists have a duty to themselves and their clients to explore their own sexuality and to feel fully comfortable with all aspects of it in order to illuminate and work through 'blind spots' which will otherwise sabotage their work. If they do not, it is highly likely that at some stage the client will find the therapist acting insincerely or even dishonestly by appearing to accept the client's homosexuality whilst disowning their *own* homosexual component.

2 *'Consider very carefully before entering into a psychotherapeutic contract to eliminate homosexual feelings and behaviour in your client. Willingness to enter into such a contract implies that homosexuality is pathological and undesirable.'* The American psychoanalyst Richard Isay, in discussing his clinical experience of patients who have 'failed' in their attempts to become heterosexual, states: 'there may be severe emotional and social consequences in the attempt to change from homosexuality to heterosexuality' (1986: 112). In speaking of the methods used by analysts who contract to facilitate this change he states:

'In each patient, the transference wish to be loved had been used by an analyst to attempt to change the patient's sexual orientation' (1986: 117). There can be grave implications for the psychological well-being of the client. The ethical considerations, raised in the previous chapter, are explored further below.

3 *'All gay people have experienced some form of oppression related to their being gay. The subjective reality of that experience must be brought into consciousness so that it can be worked with.'* Some gay clients will have no difficulty remembering anti-gay jokes and violence; however, others may report never having encountered any anti-gay oppression themselves. This may be because (a) they don't recognize anti-gay jokes as such, (b) they deliberately cultivate an ultra-heterosexual image which seeks to protect them from personal assaults or (c) they collude intra-psychically with such oppression.

4 *'Help your client to identify incorporated stereotypes of gay people and begin deprogramming and undoing the negative conditioning associated with these stereotypes.'* In an article in Gay Times, Mark Simpson (1992) attacks both the stereotypes of Straight Acting and Nelly Acting. The exaggerated hypermasculinity of the straight acting gay man is designed to 'woo the straight man and convince him that not all queers are queer'. However in playing this role, the straight acting man is playing a role just as negative as the effeminate, camp 'queen'. Simpson (1992: 54) goes on:

> Granted the 'queen' is having more fun, but it is a fun that is designed to trivialise everything, including themselves: 'Oh, don't mind me! I'm just a mad bitch!'; their souls are permanently dragged up and their hearts eternally bewigged and all emotion is mimed. Nothing will ever be sincerely experienced or expressed.

Both of these stereotypes are ways of avoiding facing up to and integrating the client's homosexuality into their general identity. Similar examples could be given for lesbians and, whilst the cultural stereotypes are to some extent time limited and therefore subject to change, for the foreseeable future there will be negative stereotypes of lesbian, gay and bisexual people. See Sinfield (1994) for an historical survey of some of them.

The aim of such work in therapy is to help the client develop an identity that is personally meaningful, and not just based on responding to heterosexual assumptions and prejudices.

5 *'While working toward expanding the range and depth of awareness of feelings, be particularly alert to facilitate the identification and expression of anger. It is helpful for the anger to be constructively channelled, and affection, openly given.'* Years of suppressing emotions can lead to male and female clients being out of touch with their feelings.

The anger generated in a punitive environment and the anger at the self for being different seem unjustified and is sent out of awareness where it continues to accumulate. Other feelings are also thus affected through generalization processes and are given less awareness or attention (Clark 1987: 219–20).

This is familiar to therapists working with men generally, and may be more common working with gay men, who have been forced to shut off their sexual–affectional world. Jourard (1971) discusses the 'lethal' effects of such masculine 'dispiritation' (see Chapter 5).

One of the known effects of denied anger, repressed pain and internalized oppression is self-abuse through the misuse of drugs, including alcohol. Another is suicide. Clark points out that the former is constantly reinforced because bars are one of the few 'community approved' meeting places for gay people and that 'suicide is implicitly encouraged by the [wider] community's failure to recognize the existence of "respectable" gay people' (1987: 222). Chapter 11 of this book discusses particular issues relating to alcohol and other drug misuse for lesbian and gay clients and Chapter 12 looks at partner abuse, often a way of 'acting out' repressed rage.

Depression is a major problem for gay people. Again, Clark sees that this results from denial of anger, denial of self-validation and 'emotional fatigue'. Being 'invisible', lesbians, gay men and bisexuals can be assaulted daily with attacks on character and ability, in 'jokes' and homophobic statements or in forms of omission of their life experience. The deep hurts are minimized, keeping anger (often with friends or family) out of awareness (Clark 1987: 220–1).

> You feel decreasing self-esteem in the uphill fight against subtle everyday messages that tend to invalidate you, and turn your anger inward on yourself. It is an unfortunate downward spiral that does not permit corrective evidence from experience.
> (Clark 1987: 130)

Working with safe, contained 'anger rituals' can prove extremely effective in moving clients away from depression and suicidal or self-harming tendencies and towards developing affirming interactions with others (see, for example, Lindenfield 1993).

6 '*Actively support appreciation of the body-self and body impulses. Don't be afraid to touch your client as a means of demonstrating that you value and trust physical contact.*' We live in a very anti-touch society, and therapists have rightly been cautioned about touching clients. However, many lesbians and gay men have grown up afraid of their bodies. Society has given them powerful messages about their bodily impulses being perverted, sick, dangerous and, specifically, a message that their feelings will be out of control. By being prepared to

Towards a model of gay affirmative therapy 33

touch clients – even a hand on the shoulder when they leave – the therapist is saying that they trust and accept the client and their body. It can be particularly healing for many gay men to be so accepted by a male therapist, when all physical contact with men has been sexualized in the past. Clark (1987: 238) says:

> Some therapists say all the right words of appreciation and never touch a client more than to shake hands. No matter how sophisticated your client or how profound the theoretical explanation of this stance, there is a primitive person inside the client who is recording a primitive message: 'If you really thought I was attractive, instead of just giving me some words to make me feel better you would want to touch me and you would find a way to touch me no matter what your ethics and training.'

Obviously, any touching should be done with ethical integrity. I am well aware of the incidence of therapists abusing clients, and would want any therapist to have clearly worked out whose needs they are serving by the touch, and to seek their clients' permission prior to each time they touch them (Rutter 1990; Russell 1993).

7 *'Encourage your client to establish a gay support system, a half-dozen gay people with mutual personal caring and respect.'* This can be particularly helpful, as creating a 'chosen family' can affirm and support the lesbian, gay or bisexual person. It is helpful to encourage friendships which go beyond, or are outside, the sexual attraction which is often the first point of contact for male relationships. Coyle (1994) notes how the mental health needs of young gay people are improved through contact with other lesbians and gay men.

8 *'Support consciousness raising efforts such as gay rap groups, pro-gay reading and involvement in gay community activities.'* ('Rap' in this context means discussion groups, rather than its current 'music' connection!) This is another way to help undo the damage of negative stereotyping of lesbian, gay and bisexual people, and help to provide competent role models of ordinary people working together for mutual benefit. The client may feel alone and wrong and fear further lack of support and affection if she or he reveals true thoughts, feelings and identity. It is unfortunate that lesbian, gay and bisexual people have to go to extra lengths to create the 'normal' sort of relationships enjoyed by many heterosexuals with their neighbours, friends and colleagues.

9 *'Work toward a peer relationship with your client. The message: you are not a second class or inferior person.'* This is crucial to gay affirmative therapy and has been elaborated throughout the previous section on core conditions of respect, so will not be expanded here.

10 *'Encourage your client to question basic assumptions about being gay and to develop a personally relevant value system as a basis for*

self-assessment. Point out the dangers of relying on society's value system for self-validation.' One of the ways in which I have found this to be helpful is in considering attitudes and values about personal relationships. The only acceptable model of sexual relationships reinforced by the state, the Church and other societal institutions is one of lifelong, or at least serial, monogamy. However, it is a model which does not appear to be very successful if we consider the rising divorce rate and surveys of infidelity. It is helpful to encourage clients to think about what they want from a relationship and why, and then to develop relationships which seek to meet their needs rather than take on unquestioningly the values of an oppressive and discriminatory society (see Chapter 6). The gradual dissociation from one's own spiritual part which results from the experience of rejection and oppression from contact with 'spiritual', religious or moral structures in society, causes deep psychological and spiritual damage, as discussed in Chapter 13.

11 *'Desensitize shame and guilt surrounding homosexual thoughts, feelings and behavior.'* In doing so, you are attempting to remove some of the power attached to the guilt and shame about being lesbian or gay. Many lesbian and gay clients feel guilty or ashamed of their sexual and affectional feelings, which they have learned to mistrust from early environmental messages that same sex attraction is bad or wrong. By warmly encouraging clients to talk about their feelings of attraction to others, you can help to break down the negative associations of same sex love. The profound effects of living with homophobia and heterosexism are discussed in the next chapter.

> Your primary objective should be to help the person to become more truly themselves, which means among other things, that you want to help the person become more truly gay, developing conscious self-appreciation and integrity that includes the integration of gay thoughts and feelings. You will not encourage self-destructive behavior and attitudes or encourage conformity, *per se*. You will instead seek to reinforce integrity by encouraging behavior and attitudes that match inner feelings.
>
> (Clark 1987: 221)

12 *'Use the weight of your authority to affirm homosexual thoughts, behavior and feelings when reported by your client.'* This is important to counteract experience of disapproval from authority figures. Whilst you have more power than your client, and assuming you are moving towards the peer relationship outlined earlier, then by warmly encouraging them to share their homosexual thoughts and feelings with you, you afford the client an experience of 'good parenting' or positive regard which has often been missing in the process of 'coming out' (see Chapter 4). Sharing their lives with someone who is encouraging is

experienced by clients as a very important facet of gay affirmative therapy. Remember that cultural promotion of conformity and discrimination against difference leads clients to feel devalued and worthless internally, however successful and accomplished outwardly.

The therapist as educator

One of the roles of gay affirmative therapy is, as with any special population, to help facilitate and educate through raising awareness. Feminist therapy makes this explicit – the role of the therapist as teacher. I have found it helpful to offer clients differing levels of information either about the process they are engaged in – for example, the stages of coming out – or about more general matters, such as lesbian or gay community issues. This educative function can:

1 provide reassurance that the client is going through a normative experience;
2 help make sense of some of their feelings, and inspire hope in a resolution;
3 delineate some of the developmental tasks necessary for a healthy integration of sexual identity into the wider personality structure.

Bibliotherapy

I have found bibliotherapy useful here. Kus (1989) describes bibliotherapy as 'the use of literature of any type, and in any form, for the purpose of self-help or personal growth'. Certain articles or books (or videos) can provide information, a diversity of affirmatory role models and something which can place the individual's experience into a wider lesbian, gay or bisexual social context.

The books I would recommend vary according to the client's needs but would include fiction as well as non-fiction. There is a power to the written word which can lend additional authority or affirmation to the work taking place in therapy. Furthermore, bibliotherapy is a cost-effective way of hastening the therapeutic process, since there is some work that the client can do on their own, and which can be reviewed in the therapeutic context.

Integrating HIV awareness into clinical practice

A further way in which the therapist can be an educator is through exploration of the client's feelings around adopting safer sex behaviours. Shernoff (1989) believes that counsellors and therapists are perfectly placed to help clients make the changes that are necessary to avoid HIV transmission.

The therapeutic relationship is characterized by unconditional respect and warmth. In this context, clients can be encouraged to explore their knowledge and fears about HIV. Health educators have clearly demonstrated that information alone is insufficient to effect prolonged behavioural change, and that two other factors are critical: (a) that someone believes themself to be at risk, and so feelings, attitudes and perceptions of risk need to be addressed, and (b) the person has the skills necessary to effect behavioural change. These skills include an ability to negotiate with sexual partners, which involves having good enough self-esteem to feel their life is worth protecting, and the skills required in condom usage. Shernoff maintains that we have an ethical duty to raise the issue of safer sex with all our clients regardless of their sexuality and I would suggest this is especially relevant when working with gay and bisexual clients, for whom there are special aspects.

Some therapists are reluctant to introduce their own issues to the agenda, and feel that it is inappropriate for them to ask clients about any issue, not least one concerning sexual behaviour. Two reasons that are often given for this, are that it is unethical for therapists to pursue a line of enquiry of their own and that, in raising such questions, the therapeutic relationship may be damaged.

It seems important to remind therapists that they are often following up issues of their own. For example, if a client mentions they are feeling totally hopeless, and wonder what the point is in living, many therapists would enquire about suicidal ideation. To avoid the issue could mean that the therapist is missing a vital clue in helping a client face fears about life and death. The majority of people who commit suicide mention it to others, albeit indirectly, before taking their lives. If a client is discussing relationships, attraction, sexuality issues, then it seems to me highly appropriate to enquire about what they are doing to protect themselves and their partners against the risk of HIV. It is disingenuous to deny that therapists are always giving information about their values, whether this is explicit or not; it is indeed the premise of this book that positive values should be communicated to clients.

As far as the second issue is concerned – the potential damage to the therapeutic relationship of raising the subject of HIV awareness – Shernoff (1989: 77) says:

> Questions of this kind often provoke profound feelings on the part of the client; these may include intense anger and sometimes relief. Anger may arise because any discussion of the subject of AIDS may challenge the client's denial and demonstrate that the therapist believes it is a relevant issue. Anger can also derive from transferential issues if the client perceives the questions as negative parental injunctions. An exploration of these negative transferential feelings can provide a fertile

ground for discussions of sex and sexuality in general, taking care of oneself, self-image and the consequences of impulsive behavior. When relief is expressed, it is most often due to the feeling that this highly charged issue can be discussed openly at last.

Therefore it can be seen that there can be a number of positive outcomes from raising the issue. However, Shernoff warns that therapists need to be familiar with HIV transmission and prevention issues and be aware of the variety of human sexual practices, as well as confident in speaking explicitly about sexual matters, which may require further training. Misinformation, or the transmission of prejudiced ideas about sexual behaviours, will be more damaging than no work around these topics.

Ethical issues

One ethical issue specifically relating to therapy with lesbian, gay and bisexual clients which needs to be addressed is whether you should accept a client into therapy who wants you to change their sexual orientation to heterosexuality. Discussion in Chapter 1, as well as that dealing with Clark's guidelines above, should have clarified the position for those wishing to offer all clients a respectful environment in which to work. Will therapists respecting a client's integrity ever contract to 'change' fundamental aspects of the client's personality? Is it ethical to treat a condition which is not an illness, but which society condemns? These questions are vital for therapists of all theoretical orientations. As we have seen in preceding pages, any therapy model which is gay affirmative (or person affirmative, in the opinion of the editors) cannot condone agreements of this nature.

Some therapists feel that if the client demands help to change their orientation, it is wrong not to respect their wish to change, and patronizing to assume they do not know their own mind. Silverstein (1977) states that no patient is 'voluntary' for sexual orientation change. They are suffering from severe problems of extreme lowering of self-esteem and significant levels of guilt;

> his [sic] request for sexual orientation change is a request for the therapist to play the role of the punishing sadist. His request is for a formally defined sadomasochistic relationship, with his playing the role of the humiliated and the therapist punishing him for transgressing the rules.
>
> (Silverstein 1977: 207)

Furthermore, Davison (1978) states that even the availability of change of orientation programmes or 'conversion' therapies (see Chapter 1) causes hurt and damage to individuals in and outside of therapy.

There has been little research on the negative effects of therapy with lesbians and gay men. Most of the major studies concerned with change of sexual orientation do not consider the negative effects of failed attempts to change on the client's self-esteem, nor do they report follow-ups on those who drop out of therapy. 'Therapies which utilize pathological models of homosexuality cannot be assumed to be helpful or even innocuous' (Cohen and Stein 1986: 20). Therapists who work in this way are acting as agents of social control and psychological manipulation. Mosher (1991: 199) also recommends political action as an ethical responsibility of helping professionals to counteract institutionalized heterosexism:

> Psychologists, as scientists and professionals committed to promoting human welfare, have a duty to end racism, sexism and heterosexism ... The straight psychotherapist's usual commitment to caring must include an unusual commitment to justice for sexual minorities if he or she is to be an effective therapist with gay men and lesbian women living in our unjust world.

Challenging heterosexism is something that all therapists should be concerned about, whether it is amongst friends and family members or one's colleagues, or within larger institutional structures.

Sexual orientation of the therapist

I believe that sexual orientation is relatively unimportant in the choice of an appropriate therapist. What is important is the therapist's ability to empathize with and accept the client. To be able to empathize fully, the therapist needs to be able to set aside their own fears and prejudices; to do this they need to be able to understand the roots of them. For an interesting account of how one heterosexual male therapist did this see Mosher (1991). It is vital that all therapists working with lesbian, gay and bisexual clients have closely examined their own heterosexism, in the same way that they have an ethical duty to be aware of, and work on, their own sexism and racism (see also Young 1995b).

One way of developing greater understanding of, and empathy with, lesbians and gay men is for the therapist to increase social contacts with lesbians and gay men. For those therapists working with a number of lesbian and gay clients perhaps participation in large-scale celebrations, such as the annual Gay Pride March, might be a useful way of demonstrating support and solidarity as well as giving an opportunity to witness the enormous diversity of lifestyles that exist.

Developing self-respect in a heterosexist world that denies respect is a major therapeutic goal in helping lesbians and gay men. A non-gay therapist may be of particular help to some clients in that the respect of the therapist, as a representative of the 'in group', can help to heal the wounds of heterosexism. Just as genuine respect and concern from a non-gay therapist can help foster self-respect it is equally important to be aware that therapists may be seen as authority figures whose (dis)approval carries much weight. They are likely to be seen as representatives of wider society, whose reactions may help the client anticipate the reactions of others in their life. 'Out' lesbian, gay and bisexual therapists may also serve as role models for clients. As Sophie (1988: 54) states 'All of these add extra weight to the therapeutic relationship and pose special challenges for the therapist.'

Heterosexual therapists need to be careful about casual references to their spouses or children, which can be experienced as indirect reminders of the therapist's 'safe' heterosexuality. This disclosure of orientation also needs to be considered by lesbian, gay and bisexual therapists who may, when working in non-gay identified settings, reveal their homosexuality on impulse without thinking through the transference and counter-transference implications; this could, for example, be experienced by the client as a seductive move.

Clients may wonder about the therapist's orientation. The meaning of this can be explored and the therapist make a clinical judgement about whether to directly reveal their sexuality, since clients may not be ready to hear it at that time. However, therapists who refuse to self-disclose in response to a direct request can cause clients to mistrust them and this can also greatly impair the therapeutic work. Sophie (1988: 56) states 'The client has a right to know, if she so wishes, whether the therapist has experienced the process of coming to terms with a non-heterosexual identity.' Therapists are reminded to consider why the client wants the information, and to explore the meaning of their response. If you are lesbian, gay or bisexual, withholding information about your orientation may be seen as an agreement with societal pressures to keep one's orientation secret (Stein 1988) (see Appendix 1).

Conclusions

This chapter presents a gay affirmative framework which is intended to augment the therapist's existing theoretical model. The guidelines given by Clark (1987) should take precedence over any theoretical constructs which run counter to them. The psychoanalytic 'blank screen' of the therapist withholding information to facilitate transference, for example, should not be held at the cost of honesty within the relationship. Nor will Rogers's (1951) 'core conditions' be adequate by themselves for humanistic practitioners because the experience of living with a stigmatized identity makes lesbian, gay and bisexual experience different from heterosexual experience (just as the experience of being black in a dominantly white and racist culture is different).

- Gay affirmative therapists are those whose beliefs and values appreciate homosexuality – and bisexuality – as valid and rich orientations in their own right and who perceive *homophobia,* not diverse sexualities, as pathological.
- Such therapists offer clients respect for their sexuality, personal integrity, culture and lifestyle.
- Therapists need (re)training to work with bi- and homosexual client groups to explore and validate their own diverse sexual feelings; to examine and address their own attitudes towards these issues; to increase awareness and understanding of such therapeutic issues as homophobia, coming out, same sex relationships; and to deepen understanding of constructions of human sexuality.
- Therapists need to remain alert to their own power and how they use this to reinforce negative authoritative messages, or to heal through self-affirming 'reparenting'. They will use supervision and personal therapy to monitor their own responses to sexual diversity.
- Therapists have a key role as educators – of other professionals with regard to sexual diversity, homophobia and mental health, as well as with clients – for example, through bibliotherapy and safer sex education.

3 | DOMINIC DAVIES

Homophobia and heterosexism

Definitions

This chapter seeks to explore one of the central clinical themes in working with lesbian, gay and bisexual clients – that of homophobia. However, it seems important to clarify a number of terms first. Weinberg (1972) is usually credited with the invention of the word, although it was in fact first coined by Smith (1971). However, it is Weinberg's (1972: 4) definition which forms the basis for most discussion and understanding of the term and the one we begin with: 'the dread of being in close quarters with homosexuals – and in the case of homosexuals themselves, self-loathing.' This definition was extended by Hudson and Ricketts (1980) to include the feelings of anxiety, disgust, aversion, anger, discomfort and fear that some heterosexuals experience around lesbians and gay men. It is this expanded meaning that will be used for the rest of this chapter and generally throughout this book.

It is important to note that the term *homophobia* has not received widespread acceptance within the literature. A number of researchers have criticized it as inaccurate, claiming that it is not a classic phobia. Other terms offered have been: *homoerotophobia* (Churchill 1967); *homosexophobia* (Levitt and Klassen 1974); *homosexism* (Lehne 1976); *homonegativism* (Hudson and Ricketts 1980); and *shame due to heterosexism* (Neisen 1990). Herek (1991) objects to the continued use of homophobia because of its tendency to pathologize the individual rather than seeing those holding anti-gay attitudes as reflecting cultural values; he prefers the use of *anti-gay prejudice*.

Whilst at a social level the term anti-gay prejudice is acceptable, it has been demonstrated (Freund *et al.* 1973; Langevin *et al.* 1975; Shields and Harriman 1984) that many individuals do exhibit a fear response to homosexuality and, whilst the origins of that fear may well be culturally derived, since it affects some people more than others there is perhaps good reason to view it in some ways as an individual anomaly. I therefore believe there is good reason to continue to use the term *homophobia*, although at times I will use *anti-gay* where that seems more contextually appropriate.

I will also be exploring the differences between *internalized homophobia* – which arises when gay men, lesbians or bisexuals themselves fear and loathe homosexuality – and *institutionalized homophobia* – in which social structures discriminate against lesbian, gay and bisexual people. This is also known as *heterosexism*: 'the system by which heterosexuality is assumed to be the only acceptable and viable life option' (Blumenfeld and Raymond 1988: 244) or to be superior or more natural.

Biphobia may be described as a fear of, and prejudice towards, bisexuals. This is sometimes used to describe the anti-bisexual sentiment of some lesbians and gay men as the objections of heterosexuals are directed towards the homosexual component of a bisexual's identity and can therefore be seen as homophobia. The term biphobia is sometimes confused with the holding of a rigid view of human sexuality allowing only two, fixed and 'opposite' orientations (hetero- and homosexual) or identities (masculine and feminine). This is more accurately defined as bipolar thinking and is not itself phobic.

Finally, definitions of more general terms: the seminal definitions of *prejudice* and *discrimination* were created by Gordon Allport (1954) in his study of racial prejudice. Unfortunately, they are just as valid more than 40 years later:

> *Prejudice* is an antipathy based on a faulty and inflexible generalization. It may be felt or expressed. It may be directed toward a group as a whole or toward an individual because he [*sic*] is a member of that group.
>
> (Allport 1954: 9)
>
> *Discrimination* comes only when we deny to individuals or groups of people equality of treatment which they may wish.
>
> (Allport 1954: 51)

The functions of prejudice

An important starting point is the examination of why homophobia exists. What purpose does it serve and why do people continue to perpetuate lies about lesbians, gays and bisexuals?

One reason could be that male homosexuality in particular is seen as a threat to the central social structure which ensures that men and 'masculine' values are dominant – patriarchy. Gay men are seen as opting out of patriarchy (Weinberg 1972) and as 'unmanly'. The negative connotations given to this term – and to 'effeminate' – are revealing in themselves. It is not uncommon for the police to boost arrest records by persecuting gay men through surveillance and prosecutions for cottaging and cruising which, by and large, are 'victimless crimes' between consenting adults, or raiding gay bars and, more recently, the private parties and homes of gay men. It would be unusual for the police to treat lesbians in this way, which led a lesbian social work educator to comment, 'It would seem that a sexual act lacks social significance unless a penis is involved' (Bernard 1992: 27).

Some psychological reasons for maintaining prejudice have been identified by Herek (1991). One of the most common is for the prejudiced person to bolster up self-esteem at the expense of oppressing the other group; for example, the evangelical Christian denouncing homosexuality in order to affirm his religious identity, or someone telling an anti-gay joke to gain the approval of their friends. It is simple to reinforce identification with 'us' by attacking 'them' (polarizing). A second function of prejudice is that, in order to make sense of a contradictory and confusing world, it is common to put people into categories, and then have a form of relating to that category. Stereotypes are one means by which people try to order their world and they provide a short cut through which people can relate to each other.

The final reason relates to resolving personal inadequacies or conflicts. For example, by scapegoating lesbian, gay and bisexual people, some heterosexuals hide from their own fears or feelings of inferiority. It is perhaps for this reason that the gay basher's violent attack serves to prop up his own fragile sense of masculinity (and heterosexuality?). Another example of this protective function would be that by constantly linking homosexuality with paedophilia, heterosexuals can distract attention from the fact that 95 per cent of child sexual abuse is perpetrated by heterosexuals. In both instances the persecutors dissociate from unacceptable feelings in themselves by projecting them onto others and then attacking them for possessing them – classic phobic processes.

Allport (1954) identified a scale of prejudice, each stage increasing the intensity of the one before it, and for our purposes it would look like this:

1 *verbal rejection* (openly verbalizing dislike of lesbian, gay and bisexual people; cracking anti-gay jokes; use of derogatory terms e.g. bum boy, lezzie, poof, batty man, etc.);
2 *discrimination* (denying equality of treatment to lesbian, gay and bisexual people; for example, in education, employment, housing, etc.);
3 *physical attack* (gay bashing and murders; rape of lesbians and gay men).

Portrait of a homophobe

Herek (1984) in a review of the literature on negative reactions to lesbians and gay men noted that some consistent patterns emerged. A person holding negative attitudes is:

1 less likely to have had personal contact with identified lesbians and gay men;
2 less likely to report having engaged in homosexual behaviours or to identify themselves as lesbian or gay;
3 more likely to perceive their peers as manifesting negative attitudes, especially if the respondents are males;
4 more likely to have resided in areas where negative attitudes are the norm, especially during adolescence;
5 likely to be older and less well educated;
6 more likely to be religious, attend church frequently, and subscribe to a conservative religious ideology;
7 more likely to express traditional, restrictive attitudes about gender roles;
8 less permissive sexually or manifesting more guilt or negativity about sexuality;
9 more likely to manifest high levels of authoritarianism and related personality characteristics.

Herek (1984) also found that heterosexuals who were homophobic had more negative attitudes to members of their own gender, and men had both stronger and deeper attitudes than women.

Institutionalized homophobia

Society has a number of different ways of discriminating against lesbian, gay and bisexual people. These structures are absorbed into the functioning of heterosexual society and serve not only to oppress lesbians, gays and bisexuals, but also to lock heterosexual men and women into rigid gender roles and self-oppressive stereotypes (see Blumenfeld 1992 for a more detailed explanation of this point).

The most common assumption underpinning these structures is that everyone else is heterosexual. Job application forms ask about 'marital status'; radio disc jockeys ask callers whether they have an 'opposite' sex girl or boyfriend and one's next of kin is expected to be a marriage partner or family member. Rarely does society take any cognizance of the fact that these situations do not apply to a sizeable minority of the population, and this serves to reinforce feelings of being excluded and of personal inadequacy. Blumenfeld (1992) cites the theologian Tinney (1983) who lists seven overlapping ways in which society oppresses lesbian, gay and bisexual people:

1 *The conspiracy of silence*: Whilst not actually enshrined in law, our society attempts to keep large numbers of lesbian, gay and bisexual people from meeting and socializing, and from open debate of the issues which affect their lives. Note, for example, the general absence of community centres and of constructive television and radio programmes about lesbian, gay and bisexual issues.
2 *The denial of culture*: History has been rewritten to exclude positive references to homosexuality and the contributions made by homo- and bisexual artists, philosophers, composers, etc. Boswell (1980) has documented numerous examples of this through censorship, deletion, half-truths, and the changing of gender pronouns.
3 *The denial of popular strength*: No matter how many sex surveys show the incidence of homosexual behaviour or identity, the general population (aided by the media) continues to deny the existence of lesbian, gay and bisexual people. It has been over 45 years since Kinsey *et al.* (1947) reported that 37 per cent of males had at least one sexual experience to orgasm with another man during their adult life. Yet still lesbians, gays and bisexuals are denied equality of treatment and their civil rights in Britain and in many places in the world. For example, it took a serial killer on the streets of London at around the time of the Gay Pride March in 1993 for the media to cover what had been for the previous three years the largest civil rights event or festival in London's crowded calendar of marches (in 1994 approximately 160,000 attended the festival). The mainstream press had always chosen to ignore it. When homosexuality is covered, it is usually trivialized or implies that lesbians, gays and bisexuals live in some seedy, twilight world of promiscuity, violence and danger. The reader is invited to examine their own newspapers and magazines for anti-gay bias.
4 *Fear of over-visibility*: Some heterosexuals, and even some homosexuals, feel uncomfortable with open discussions of same sex attractions and relationships. It is seen as normal for a heterosexual to discuss how they spent their weekend, but if a gay man shares information about his weekend, some people would say he was 'flaunting' his homosexuality. The message is 'I don't care what you do in private, but don't force your homosexuality down my throat.' It could be said that 'good gays' are those who are quiet about their lives. Many people still have great difficulty discussing homosexuality and use euphemisms to avoid saying what they mean: 'He's that way'; 'She's very manly.'
5 *Creation of defined public spaces*: Society often prefers ghettos for gay spaces. In Britain, for example, this would include the 'gay villages' of Old Compton Street in Soho, London or around Bloom Street in Manchester. The concept of social space need not necessarily be geographical. The annual Lesbian and Gay Pride March through central London in June means that these communities feel safe to express affection in

public – for one day a year the law regarding 'behaviour likely to cause a breach of the peace' is ignored.

6 *Denial of self-labelling*: Lesbians and gay men have chosen those terms to define themselves as a more positive way to describe themselves. Gay men continue to be referred to by many people as homosexuals which the majority of them find offensive. Terms of abuse (queer, poof, dyke, and lezzie) are commonly used against anyone who is unpopular or despised regardless of their sexuality, and are often unchallenged by parents and teachers. Recently some sections of the lesbian and gay communities have been reappropriating terms such as queer, faggot and dyke to neutralize their hate value and challenge their negative meaning:

> Nothing makes liberals – gay and straight – squirm more than calling yourself queer. It reminds them of the degree to which they ignore homophobia every day by talking about 'gay' people. Straights think they've done everything we've demanded by simply changing the language they use to patronise us.
> (Queer Nation activist quoted by Alcorn 1992: 75)

7 *Negative symbolism*: Heterosexual society lays down norms and rules of behaviour from which minority groups are seen to deviate. These differences are then seen as inadequacies on the part of the minority group to 'make the grade'. Stereotypes are created to enshrine deviant identities in those who have different values. An example of this is how lesbians and gays are excluded from the legal and social privileges of marriage, then ascribed traits of lacking commitment to relationships, inability to be intimate, and living highly promiscuous lifestyles. In doing this, society projects its shadow side onto minority groups. Long ago black people were stereotyped as evil practitioners of voodoo and black magic, because some of their forms of spirituality were unlike the traditional quiet worship of Christianity. Lesbians and gay men are stereotyped as having no control over their sexual desires, leading them to be promiscuous, dangerous to be around (because they will always be making passes), child molesting hedonists trying to recruit others into a homosexual lifestyle. (These ideas led some gay activists to parody this absurdity and wear T shirts with the message: 'Bring us your children, what we don't fuck, we'll eat!'.)

Institutionalized homophobia in society

The presumption of heterosexuality and the discrimination that results from institutionalized homophobia can lead to oppression in a number of key areas. Oppression can be seen to follow a cycle (Walsh 1992). The

Figure 1 Cycle of oppression

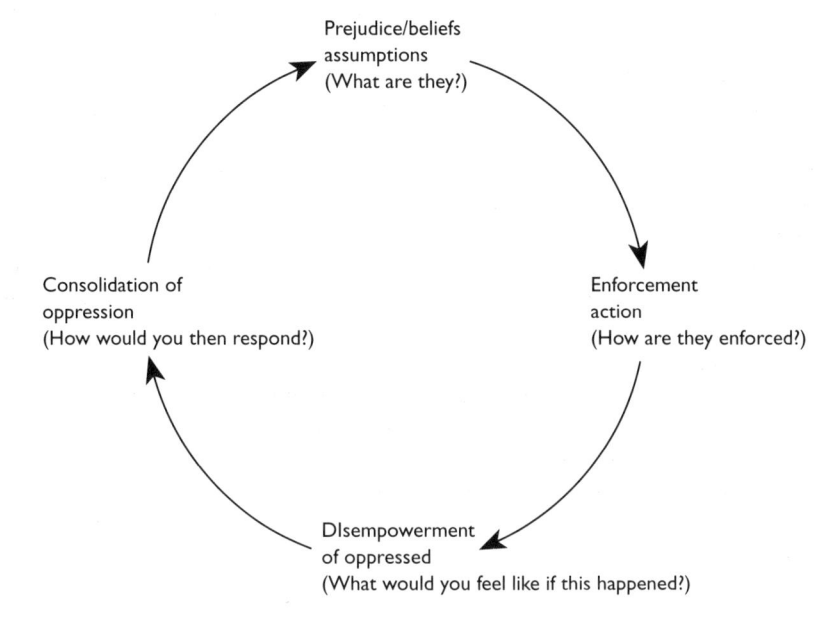

```
                    Prejudice/beliefs
                    assumptions
                    (What are they?)


  Consolidation of                          Enforcement
  oppression                                action
  (How would you then respond?)             (How are they enforced?)


                    Disempowerment
                    of oppressed
                    (What would you feel like if this happened?)
```

Source: © Fran Walsh, February 1992 Reproduced with kind permission

reader may find it helpful to brainstorm words, images and feelings that come to mind for each of the four categories in Figure 1.

I propose to explore just three areas where homophobia has become institutionalized: education, leisure and employment; there are many more. The interested reader could follow up with some of the reading suggested in Appendix 3.

Education

Schools are often worried about teaching about homosexuality, lest they be charged under Section 28 of the Local Government Act 1990 which forbids 'the promotion of homosexuality as a pretend family relationship'. Many schools self-censor as a result of this, and are anxious about being seen to encourage positive images of lesbian, gay and bisexual people (see Rivers 1995a, 1995b). However, the government also removed power from the local education authorities to decide what should be taught under sex education, giving it instead to school governors. This could mean that, with liberal governors, positive images of homosexuality could be finding their way into classrooms.

Why is it important to include positive images of homosexuality in the classroom? First, in order to reassure young people who know they are, or think they may be, lesbian, gay or bisexual that their sexuality is natural and healthy. Second, to educate heterosexual young people about sexual and cultural diversity in order to break down homophobia and heterosexism and free them from oppressive stereotypes and bipolar thinking. Third, to help those unsure about their sexuality by giving accurate and honest information about sexual diversity, so that they can find support for themselves and make up their own minds with the minimum of fear, denial and oppression. Finally, given that they have a much neglected cultural identity and history of their own, to help lesbian, gay and bisexual students, in particular, learn about their culture in the same way that Afro-Caribbean young people are now learning about themselves. It is just as important that all students learn something about the larger minority cultural groups in our society.

This is why it would be helpful to have openly lesbian, gay and bisexual teachers who could provide positive role models and support to students. It would also be helpful when studying a topic to know whether the person studied was lesbian, gay or bisexual to further one's understanding of the issues. Further discussion of educational issues will be found in Chapter 8.

Leisure

Sports
The ethos of sports centres, especially changing rooms and team sports, remind many lesbian, gay and bisexual people of the intimidation and fear they experienced at school, and so are avoided. Male team sports are usually heterosexually dominated and, because of the macho environment, intimidating to gay or bisexual men and boys.

Women's team sports, especially rugby and football, attract a large number of lesbians. Because of their feminist roots, there is a greater acceptance of lesbianism within women's team sports, although there is often a need to keep this covert in order that players avoid the homophobia of others connected with the sport, whether officially or unofficially; for example, homophobic male officials discriminating against women's sport, or husbands and boyfriends becoming suspicious of their female partners playing rugby every Sunday. At a higher level, it is interesting to note that the lesbianism of some champions, such as Martina Navratilova in tennis, has not reduced their success or hugely popular following.

Cinema, theatre and television
Increasingly there have been gay characters in films. Often these are negative stereotypes, from the bisexual ice-pick wielding serial killer in *Basic Instinct* to the camp gay neighbour in *Frankie and Johnnie*. For a more detailed account of lesbian and gay imagery on film see Vito Russo's *The*

Celluloid Closet (1991). It is impossible at present to find a mainstream Hollywood movie which depicts a central lesbian, gay or bisexual character positively and without resorting to stereotypes. This is clearly due to the homophobia of the Hollywood film industry. For a detailed analysis of this, one could do no better than read *Queer in America* by Michelangelo Signorile (1994).

It is in the fringe theatre and cinema where some of the greatest advances in celebrating and chronicling diverse sexual identities have been made. Plays, solo performers and low budget movies now seek to reflect lesbian, gay and bisexual lives and document our experience, culture and history.

There have also been four series of programmes made by Channel Four television aimed at the lesbian and gay communities. These programmes were vulnerable and when Channel Four had a cash crisis in 1993, the series was one of the first to be cut. It was reintroduced in 1994; although a networked national lesbian and gay television series was unique to Channel Four, it amounts only to about 10 hours' programming a year. This is not a reasonable representation given the estimated population of these communities in the UK, and considering Channel Four's specific minority broadcasting brief.

Special interest groups

The March 1996 edition of the national monthly magazine *Gay Times* (see Appendix 2) listed over 140 special interest groups. They included chamber choirs, deaf support groups, groups for people of different nationalities, sports and leisure groups. Bisexuals, lesbians and gay men can meet others to share in their hobbies and interests. However, the majority of these groups are based in London and run by and for men.

For people living outside the capital the situation can vary dramatically and, for an up to date picture of what is currently available, it would be better to call the nearest gay switchboard. A great many groups outside of London aim to provide social support to people experiencing loneliness and isolation. There are very few dedicated to providing for a genuine leisure interest, for example, gay bridge players or gardeners. It would seem the energy of provincial gay communities is still needed to provide support rather than getting on with the creation of an active social life around specific interests or leisure activities (see Chapter 5).

Employment

There are numerous examples of lesbians and gay men being discriminated against in the work place. In a relatively small, but important, survey conducted in 1986 by Lesbian and Gay Employment Rights (LAGER) (Greasley 1986), 78 per cent of the gay male respondents said they had not been open about their sexuality when applying for their current job. Out of the 200 respondents 12 had lost their jobs because they were gay and 51 had experienced trouble at work related to their gayness. These difficulties included being sacked, demoted or refused promotion. Those eligible to appeal to an employment appeals tribunal against dismissal usually found the employer's side upheld, and the appeals panel finding in favour of the employer's discrimination. This was particularly the case if the person worked with the public or with young people.

Institutionalized homophobia within the mental health professions

The mental health professions have not escaped the insidious effects of anti-gay prejudice and discrimination either. This is not surprising, since we have seen in Chapter 2 that psychiatry and psychotherapy have been responsible for some of the most appalling atrocities in the name of 'healing'. If we examine three interlinked areas – training courses, supervision and consultation and, finally, clinical practice – we can see examples of heterosexist assumptions and homophobic prejudice at work.

Training course issues

> The failure to include in professional training programs the more recent, psychologically sophisticated literature that debunks the old myths and stereotypes is the manifest expression of the [psychiatric] profession's own homophobia, maintained in the face of scientific study to the contrary.
> (Forstein 1988: 34)

The reader will recognize that it is not just the psychiatric profession that is remiss. Most British counselling and psychotherapy training programmes do not include specific input on working with lesbian, gay and bisexual clients as part of the core curriculum. To our knowledge only one BAC-recognized course has included a three day block. There are a number of implications resulting from the exclusion of this specific teaching. It will have significant impact on lesbian, gay or bisexual therapists in training. As part of the research for this chapter, I wrote to a number of lesbian, gay and bisexual therapists about their experiences in training. Here are a few examples:

> In a seminar on Relationship Counselling I said to the participants, 'You do all know I'm a lesbian don't you?' One of the other women replied; 'Oh yes X, we don't mind.'

> I found it hard to be out during the training, although when I was I found my fellow participants very positive and supportive; I'm less sure about the tutors. And I believe that affected the extent to which I felt comfortable about sharing myself and my experiences on the training modules – if you're only half-out maybe you're only half there.

A common criticism of courses was that the staff failed to recognize the political nature of homophobia and heterosexism. Often courses may have a lone lesbian, gay man or bisexual who can feel extremely isolated. Unless they challenge anti-gay prejudice, usually it won't be challenged, and sometimes they then get accused of 'banging the same old drum': 'I would have liked to have felt that heterosexism would be firmly challenged by the tutors when it occurred, and not left to more aware course participants.' It is, of course, extremely important that *all* trainees address heterosexism and homophobia regardless of their own sexual orientation.

Participants may not understand many of the issues around being *out* and lesbian, gay or bisexual.

> I was 'outed' to the whole course by a fellow participant during an angry attack. My challenge of her was not understood by staff or participants, which left me feeling more isolated than before. I came close to leaving the course.

A number of points about the importance of incorporating lesbian, gay and bisexual issues into counsellor training are made by Buhrke (1989) who states:

1 There is heterosexist bias inherent in many traditional counselling theories and theories of personality development (e.g. Freud's genital stages of development prescribe heterosexual pairing (Crain 1985) and Erikson's stages of development).
2 It is important that counsellors can discriminate when the client's sexual orientation should be the focus of counselling and when it should be left alone (e.g. if a client comes to work on her relationship, sexual orientation should not be the focus).
3 In counselling placements, counsellor trainers should give students sufficient background and knowledge about lesbian, gay and bisexual issues so that clients do not have to educate the counsellors about their lifestyles and counselling supervisors should monitor their cases for heterosexual bias or homophobia.
4 Alongside other developmental issues, trainers should include information on the development of a lesbian, gay or bisexual identity and the coming out process as well as information about lesbian and gay issues across the life span.

5 The particular differences in lesbian and gay relationships and couple counselling should be addressed, as well as issues around psychosexual dysfunction and sex therapy with lesbians and gay men.
6 Working with the families of lesbians and gay men and with young lesbian and gay clients should also be covered.

It is my contention that institutionalized prejudice is operating in most British counsellor training programmes. Courses not only fail to attract students from ethnic minorities, they also fail to address the needs of, and provide support for, the differently abled and, of course, lesbian, gay and bisexual students, as well as clients from these groups. Course staff are often exclusively white, able-bodied heterosexuals and the courses naturally attract students from these groups. Often course exercises are phrased in ways which reflect a heterosexist bias. However, if we were to accept Cayleff's point that it is unethical for us to work with culturally different clients when we have not had any training to do so (see p. 29), how many of our profession would turn away a client on this basis? Just how often is it that we are happy to take the fees of culturally different students and clients without adequately preparing ourselves to work with them? Courses may like to consider engaging an equalities consultant to review their recruitment and selection procedure, as well as to go through the course syllabus for bias.

Supervision and consultation issues

Another area where homophobia can go unchallenged is within supervision and consultation. There are two situations I wish to explore here: the supervision of heterosexual therapists by heterosexual consultants of work with lesbian, gay and bisexual clients; and the experience of being a lesbian, gay or bisexual therapist supervised by a heterosexual consultant.

Where both consultant and therapist are heterosexual there is a need for the consultant to have some training in cross-cultural issues and to be aware that they are listening through their own 'cultural filters'. This is especially relevant if either person has not had training in gay affirmative therapy and worked on their own homophobia. Tievsky (1988: 58) suggests indicators that consultants could pay attention to in watching for homophobia in the therapist:

> Some of the clues that researchers have determined as indicators of the existence of homophobia include joking about it (Gramick 1983), uneasiness (Moses and Hawkins 1982), hostility, stereotyping and denial (Messing *et al.* 1984), and exaggerating the significance of the client's orientation (Rabin *et al.* 1986), and of course pity (Woodman and Lenna 1980). Another indicator frequently found among profes-

sional psychotherapists is the attitude that sexual orientation makes absolutely no difference, thus ignoring the impact of life in a rejecting society (Messing *et al.* 1984).

Consultants and supervisors need to be scrupulous in not imposing their own (heterosexual) frame of reference onto the client. In trying to understand what might be going on in the client's life, the assumptions and interpretations concluded from the evidence may be viewed very differently by someone experienced in gay subcultural norms and values. Hopefully this book will serve as a way of educating non-gay therapists and supervisors in some of the differences experienced by lesbian, gay and bisexual people.

One of the difficulties that a lesbian, gay or bisexual therapist may experience in taking their clinical work to supervision with a non-gay consultant is of self-censoring either to protect themselves from being judged or to protect their client's life from being judged (albeit covertly).

> I was working with Mike, a 44-year-old gay man who met most of his sexual partners in cottages [public toilets]. I delayed for several sessions before taking our work to supervision because I thought my supervisor would either pathologize him as depraved, or incapable of creating 'normal' sexual relationships. I didn't want to have to get into explaining the various *ins* and *outs* of cottaging to her. I also didn't want her to know my knowledge about this came from my own experience of having met people in this way and be similarly judged.
>
> In the end I needed to raise our work in supervision and my supervisor seemed fine about it, but it did take most of the session to explain just about cottaging, before we could get near to the clinical issue I was bringing.

It is again helpful if the supervisor has had some training in lesbian and gay therapy issues *before* working with lesbian, gay and bisexual therapists, and perhaps a commitment to private reading and research, rather than expecting the therapist to explain things to them. Clearly consultants have a responsibility to work on, and be aware of, their own homophobia and heterosexism. A further example of this comes from a heterosexual consultant who supervises a gay male therapist:

> James was an out gay man with whom I have worked in supervision for some years. In the early period of our relationship when I noticed he was sometimes very tired, I had to challenge in myself from time to time the thought that he was being excessively self-regarding and that he lacked 'fibre', as my public school background would have had it. The thought was clearly related to homophobic images of 'limp

wristed queens' etc. which hardly relates to his actual self-presentation or the reality of his situation.

Clinical practice issues

There can also be issues around working with a heterosexual therapist. One lesbian client commented to me that:

> I find myself censoring what I say to my therapist; for example, I might try to avoid talking about bad experiences with men just in case she thinks 'Ah, that's why she's a lesbian.' I don't quite trust that she understands being a dyke is a positive choice for me.

This can be a difficult challenge for heterosexual therapists, the self-censoring of material by the client. The therapist may be presumed homophobic, or at least heterosexually biased, unless they are able to actively demonstrate they are keen to work on their own biases and are open to learning. This was demonstrated by the therapist of another colleague, who wrote:

> In my individual therapy with a heterosexual man . . . I can honestly say that his heterosexuality has not been anything of a barrier, nor has my gayness. He is well versed in our subcultural issues, receptive and positively encouraging me to educate him where he has no knowledge (I told him about the THT [Terrence Higgins Trust] gay safer sex video and he bought it and uses it on a sexuality course he teaches). I feel his affinity and support absolutely and he has never in any way problematized my sexuality.

High praise indeed and, hopefully, encouragement to heterosexual therapists reading this book and wondering whether they can be helpful to their lesbian, gay and bisexual clients.

It is worth bearing in mind Kinsey's 37 per cent figure for male participation in same sex sexual activity to orgasm. Many heterosexually identified men have a history that includes both homosexual activity and anti-homosexual prejudice. This may leave them feeling anxious and confused. It is important that such men understand their experiences and their feelings about them and resolve any anxieties they may have around working with homosexual and bisexual clients.

Internalized homophobia

Lesbians, gay men and bisexuals spend every day of their lives knowing that some sections of society wish they did not exist. The hatred and prejudice experienced can in some people grow like a cancer and become 'intra-psychically malignant' (Forstein 1988: 34). Internalized homophobia is a central clinical theme in working with lesbian, gay and bisexual clients. A number of therapists have written about it, and this section seeks to present some useful suggestions for understanding, identifying and responding to it.

> Negative feelings about one's sexual orientation may be over generalized to encompass the entire self. Effects of this may range from a mild tendency toward self-doubt in the face of prejudice to overt self-hatred and self-destructive behaviour.
> (Gonsiorek and Rudolph 1991: 166)

> At some point in intensive psychotherapy, every gay man expresses unhappiness and dissatisfaction with his homosexuality. The socialization of every homosexual involves internalization of the social animosity he experiences.
> (Isay 1989: 120)

It is practically impossible for a lesbian, gay or bisexual person who has grown up in British society *not* to have internalized society's negative messages about their sexuality. Whilst most people feel glad to be gay, at some, often unconscious, level there will be uneasiness with their sexuality. It is the therapist's task to uncover these self-oppressive beliefs and behaviours and, by making them conscious, assist the client to see the material as a direct result of societal pathologizing of their natural and healthy sexuality.

It is important for therapists not to be afraid to ask about the negative feelings associated with being lesbian, gay or bisexual. Offering gay affirmative therapy does not imply that the therapist should take an enthusiastically positive stance. If the enquiry occurs in the context of a trusting relationship where the client feels their sexuality is valued then it is unlikely to be experienced as an attempt to persuade someone into heterosexuality, or as homophobia on the part of the therapist. However, it is useful for therapists to be alert to the possibility of their questions being seen in that light. It is also common for people from a stigmatized group to have become so fiercely 'loyal' to that group in the face of constant attacks that they are reluctant to admit their own less positive feelings.

Therapists also need to be aware that the client may view the therapist as a representative of societal and familial prohibitions against homosexuality and therefore project a strong negative transference onto the therapist. The area of actual sexual behaviour may be particularly difficult for the lesbian or gay client to discuss, and the therapist needs to be comfortable enough to encourage openness and able to provide accurate information when needed.

Carmen de Monteflores (1986) identified four intrapsychic and interpersonal ways of coping with homophobia and heterosexism amongst 'fairly well-adjusted lesbians and gay men':

1 *Assimilation* – 'The core issue of assimilation is survival.' Assimilation is the taking on of behaviour, attitudes and language of the dominant group and thereby 'passing' as heterosexual. As a result 'there can be a profound sense of self-betrayal as well, an inner unease, a disconnection with the values of one's culture of origin' (de Monteflores 1986: 75, 76). In addition, strong feelings of anger, guilt and resentment can derive from not really being 'seen' or 'known' by others, sometimes including those most loved or cared about.
2 *Confrontation* – an example of this would be 'coming out'. By challenging negative stereotyping, one is encouraging 'the transformation of an apparent deficit into a strength' (de Monteflores 1986: 77). Coming out begins with self-affirmation and usually results in some kind of public acknowledgement of the 'new' identity. Some people express their anger at the experience of stigma by 'acting out' confrontatively when this is not appropriate (see the case example of Jamie in Chapter 8 of this book for instance).
3 *Ghettoization* – living a significant part of one's life in a geographical and/or psychological subculture. In most cities with large lesbian and gay communities, there will be certain neighbourhoods which will have a higher than average proportion of lesbians and gay men. The psychological subculture can be maintained through only socializing with other lesbians and gay men, reading only gay literature and newspapers, and socializing in exclusively gay venues. This can sometimes be accompanied by polarizing heterosexuals and their cultural norms as contemptible, or even pathological, in return! (see p. 62).
4 *Specialization* – de Monteflores (1986: 80) defines this as: 'seeing oneself as special as a function of having unique qualities, for example, being exotic, having special talents as a group, being better for having suffered or for surviving suffering and seeing oneself as belonging to a "chosen" or "exiled" group'. This is of course a defensive rationalization (see Margolies *et al.* 1987 later in this chapter).

Sophie (1988) identified six coping strategies employed by her lesbian clients coming to terms with changes in their sexual orientation. These methods were effective in dealing with internalized homophobia and could also apply to gay men and bisexuals:

1 *Cognitive restructuring* – is at the heart of eradicating or lessening internalized homophobia and forming a positive view of one's sexuality. The therapist can help by being willing to explore some of the negative stereotypes of lesbians, gay men and bisexuals and exploring the diversity

of their communities. *Bibliotherapy* (the therapeutic use of appropriate gay affirmative literature, fiction and non-fiction) can also be helpful in this process.

2 *Avoiding a negative identity* – Sophie (1985, 1988) found a difference between her non-clinical research participants and a clinical population in that many participants avoided coming out as lesbian regardless of their experience, until they felt at least neutral, if not positive about the identity label. The therapeutic usefulness of this research is that clients who are ambivalent about labelling themselves as lesbian or gay can be encouraged to keep an open mind and explore the possibilities for themselves before taking on the identity label. The researcher helpfully cautions:

> One must bear in mind the great flexibility and variety of experiences actually reported by participants in this and other research, in contrast to the dichotomous view we commonly hold of sexual orientation (see, e.g., Bell and Weinberg 1978; Shively *et al.* 1983–4). It is quite possible that the client is neither homosexual nor heterosexual, but some combination of both. This requires a sensitivity to the ambiguity and complexity of sexual orientation on the part of the therapist; both therapist and client must be able to live with this complex understanding of sexual orientation.
>
> (Sophie 1988: 58)

3 *Adopting an identity label* – by taking on a label one develops a sense of belonging to a community of interest. The support that this can generate is obviously helpful. Some previously heterosexually identified people, as they become aware of changes in their orientation and begin to relate to other lesbians or gay men, may adopt the label of bisexual. This, they believe, has less stigma attached to it, and it allows them to keep a foot in the door of heterosexual acceptability. However, homophobia amongst heterosexuals often means that bisexuals are rejected and biphobia amongst lesbians and gay men can lead to opposition because of the person's heterosexuality. Furthermore if someone delays for too long the adoption of a lesbian or gay identity, it may prevent them from making relationships within the lesbian or gay communities. Many genuine bisexuals are now able to adopt an identity label which is congruent and receive support from an increasingly organized bisexual community (see Appendix 2).

4 *Self-disclosure* – the importance of 'coming out' and declaring one's difference to the heterosexual norm to people who are important in the client's life is also a very significant strategy for dealing with internalized homophobia. The process by which this takes place is dealt with in much more detail in Chapter 4. It is worth noting here that covert internalized homophobia can lead to poorly judged disclosures with negative consequences, which further reinforce low self-esteem.

5 *Meeting other lesbian, gay and bisexual people* – this helps undermine negative stereotypes and is again a fundamental aid to cognitive restructuring. This is further developed by Sophie's (1988) final coping strategy:
6 *Habituation to homosexuality* – this is where the person's homosexuality becomes ordinary rather than unusual. Relationships with the same sex and socializing within the lesbian, gay and bisexual communities are no longer strange or different, but part of the regular experience of the person. By breaking down the barriers of unfamiliarity, the person also challenges their internalized homophobia.

Some clinical manifestations of internalized homophobia

Clients rarely seek therapy to deal with self-labelled internalized homophobia. Their homophobia is most often expressed in conjunction with other issues and remains embedded in a wide range of experiences.
(Margolies *et al.* 1987: 234)

It is unusual, although not unknown, for a client to present for therapy saying they hate themselves because they are lesbian or gay. Their internalized homophobia is more likely to come out through subtler means. For example, there is an increased prevalence of substance abuse amongst lesbians, gay men and bisexuals due to the management of living with a stigmatized identity and the fact that alcohol in particular is a socially sanctioned and freely available anxiety remover. Pubs and clubs are the most common meeting places for lesbians, gays and bisexuals to socialize (Smith 1988: 64). In examining alcohol abuse Saghir and Robins (1973) found 35 per cent of their lesbian sample and 30 per cent of their gay sample engaged in 'excessive drinking behaviour' compared with 5 per cent of heterosexual women and 20 per cent of heterosexual men in the general population. This issue is explored in greater detail by Kowszun and Malley in Chapter 11.

Other more overt examples of internalized homophobia include higher levels of depression, self-harm, and suicide attempts amongst lesbians and gay men than amongst the general population. Coyle (1993) found levels of psychological well-being amongst gay men comparable with groups from the general population who had undergone potentially traumatic life events; for example divorced, separated and widowed men.

It is not uncommon for ego defence mechanisms to operate which seek to protect the person from emotional stress, and yet which serve to alienate them from themselves. Denial may lead to emotional alienation and reaction formation – trying to become 'the best little boy in the world' in a futile attempt to prove that he is lovable – which may lead to self-neglect, loss of identity and over caretaking for others: further examples of internalized homophobia.

The training consultant Anthony Hillin has constructed Figures 2 and 3 to chart the effects of internalized homophobia (Bremner and Hillin 1993). Figure 2 shows the extent of the effect of internalized homophobia amongst gay men. Some of the elements Hillin catalogues may be due to being male, or may have other aetiology, but clinical experience suggests these issues are common to large numbers of gay men. Figure 3 offers constructive and practical advice for arresting the cycle of oppression.

Margolies and her colleagues at the Boston Lesbian Psychologies Collective (Margolies *et al.* 1987) identified eight ways in which internalized homophobia can present itself. I have set these into a clinical context by using case vignettes.

Case example 1: Fear of discovery
Sometimes it is necessary to 'pass' as heterosexual. However, some lesbians and gay men will 'pass' to protect others:

> Adam and Bob have lived together for five years. They are both successful businessmen and enjoy a comfortable lifestyle. Adam believes his family doesn't know he is gay so when his parents come to visit Bob moves into a separate bedroom and the flat is tidied up to conceal any references to homosexuality. Adam believes that coming out would be so difficult for his family to cope with and, as his father has a heart condition, he doesn't want to take the risk. His parents get on well with Bob, and Adam and Bob think his parents see them just as good house mates.

This may be an example of internalized homophobia. Adam and Bob are utilizing what psychodynamic practitioners refer to as the defence mechanisms of projection and rationalization.

Case example 2: Discomfort with obvious lesbians and gays
The 'bull dyke' or 'camp queen' image evokes public scorn and condemnation that some more 'normal-looking' lesbians and gay men feel they don't deserve:

> Colin works out at the gym three times a week, and prefers not to go out on the gay 'scene'. He is concerned not to be seen going in or coming out of local gay pubs. When he is abroad on holiday, he enjoys frequenting gay clubs, restaurants etc. but at home he feels very uneasy. There are one or two out gay men at the large firm where he works. Colin prefers not to be seen talking with them, as they are 'a bit camp and someone might start putting two and two together'.

Colin is utilizing what psychodynamic practitioners refer to as the defence mechanism of identification with the aggressor.

Figure 2 This chart shows the patterns by which gay male oppression is internalized. The mechanisms by which other oppressions are internalized are similar while the content varies

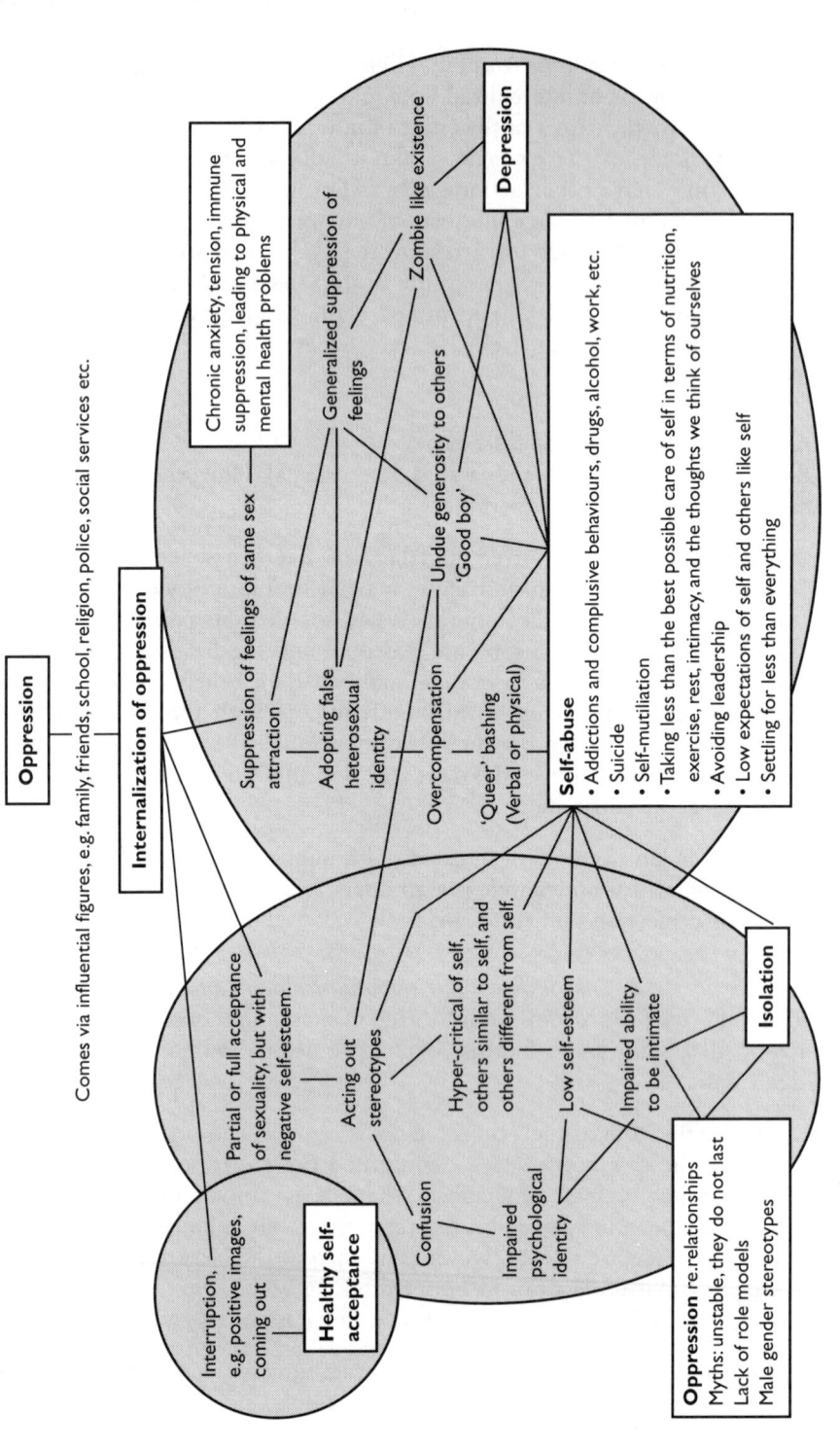

Comes via influential figures, e.g. family, friends, school, religion, police, social services etc.

Oppression

Internalization of oppression

- Suppression of feelings of same sex attraction
- Adopting false heterosexual identity
- Overcompensation
- 'Queer' bashing (Verbal or physical)
- Undue generosity to others 'Good boy'
- Generalized suppression of feelings
- Zombie like existence
- Chronic anxiety, tension, immune suppression, leading to physical and mental health problems

Depression

Self-abuse
- Addictions and compulsive behaviours, drugs, alcohol, work, etc.
- Suicide
- Self-mutilation
- Taking less than the best possible care of self in terms of nutrition, exercise, rest, intimacy, and the thoughts we think of ourselves
- Avoiding leadership
- Low expectations of self and others like self
- Settling for less than everything

Healthy self-acceptance
- Interruption, e.g. positive images, coming out
- Partial or full acceptance of sexuality, but with negative self-esteem.
- Acting out stereotypes
- Confusion
- Hyper-critical of self, others similar to self, and others different from self.
- Low self-esteem
- Impaired ability to be intimate
- Impaired psychological identity

Isolation

Oppression re.relationships
- Myths: unstable, they do not last
- Lack of role models
- Male gender stereotypes

Source: © Anthony Hillin, Training and Consultancy, 69 Pretoria Avenue, London E17 6JZ

Figure 3 Interrupting the cycle of internalized oppression

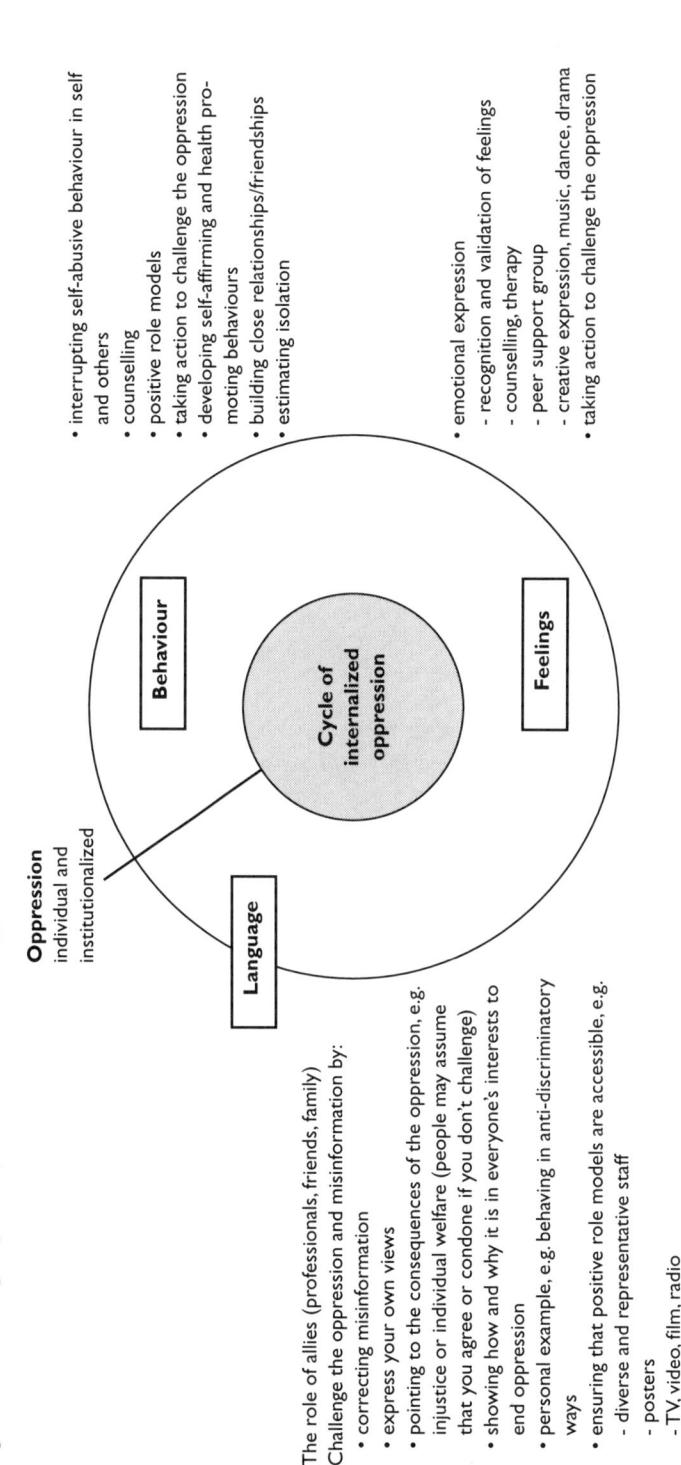

Oppression
individual and institutionalized

- interrupting self-abusive behaviour in self and others
- counselling
- positive role models
- taking action to challenge the oppression
- developing self-affirming and health promoting behaviours
- building close relationships/friendships
- estimating isolation

Behaviour

Cycle of internalized oppression

Feelings

- emotional expression
- recognition and validation of feelings
- counselling, therapy
- peer support group
- creative expression, music, dance, drama
- taking action to challenge the oppression

Language

The role of allies (professionals, friends, family)
Challenge the oppression and misinformation by:
- correcting misinformation
- express your own views
- pointing to the consequences of the oppression, e.g. injustice or individual welfare (people may assume that you agree or condone if you don't challenge)
- showing how and why it is in everyone's interests to end oppression
- personal example, e.g. behaving in anti-discriminatory ways
- ensuring that positive role models are accessible, e.g.
  - diverse and representative staff
  - posters
  - TV, video, film, radio
  - books
  - discussion
- supporting and assisting the individual's own actions.

Source: © Anthony Hillin, Training and Consultancy, 69 Pretoria Avenue, London E17 6JZ

Case example 3: Rejection and denigration of all heterosexuals (heterophobia)
By putting down or avoiding all heterosexuals one is demonstrating a reverse discrimination:

> Diane is actively involved in the lesbian community. She works as a volunteer for a lesbian line and lives in a lesbian housing co-op. She drinks in lesbian run pubs. Where possible she avoids all contact with heterosexuals and with men. She does know some heterosexual women who use the local women's centre, whom she denigrates because of their relationships with men.

Diane is using the defence mechanism of projection to try to justify her position. 'Where... homosexuality is ego-syntonic, [the person] doesn't require anyone to share [their] values and lifestyle' (Margolies *et al.* 1987: 232).

Case example 4: Feeling superior to heterosexuals
Some lesbians and gay men may exhibit an exaggerated gay pride, a false embracing of their differentness:

> Edward and Frank are both glad to be gay. *Very* glad. Edward is an actor and feels his gayness has given him an added sensitivity to human suffering. Frank works in a gay owned clothing store. He sees gay designers as being more popular, and their work more creative than clothing designed by heterosexuals.

They are both of the opinion that 'We're better because we have a harder life.' This is both a rationalization and a reaction formation response, and what cognitive therapists call dissonance reduction: if this medicine tastes so vile it *must* be doing me good.

Case example 5: Belief that lesbians and gay men are not different from heterosexuals

> Gill is a school teacher in a small suburban primary school. She lives with Hattie, her lover of 15 years. They do not socialize on the commercial gay scene but do have a number of friends, mostly heterosexual, with whom they socialize on a regular basis at each others' homes. They do not see any point in participating in their local lesbian community, nor in reading the gay press. They feel some lesbians make too much out of their sexuality, and what they do in bed is no business of anyone else's.

There is rationalization and denial operating here.

Case example 6: Uneasiness with children being raised in single-sex households
By colluding with the heterosexist myth that children need two parents of different genders, one is ignoring the many millions of households of single parent families and, as psychodynamic theorists would say, 'identifying with the aggressor'.

> Iona desperately wanted to have children, but because she felt that children needed a parent of each gender she got married. She stopped having sex with her husband immediately after the birth of her second child, and he began affairs with numerous other women, which he used to goad Iona with. She felt unable to leave him because she believed the children 'needed a father'.

Chapter 7 discusses same sex and single parenting options and acknowledges the importance of a range of 'models' of both genders being available to children.

Case example 7: Restricting attractions to unavailable people

> John is 22 and in love with his best friend Kevin, 'who happens to be straight'. They went to the same school and, during their late adolescence after getting very drunk, they 'found themselves' in bed together. They mutually masturbated and the following day Kevin denied all knowledge of the events of the previous night. Some months later, John agreed to move in with Kevin to help share the costs of a fairly heavy mortgage. John presented for counselling with severe mood swings. If Kevin was nice to him, he felt elated. If Kevin ignored him or brought home a girlfriend, John felt totally devastated. John feels that if he's patient enough, Kevin 'will sort himself out' and want to settle down with him. Kevin seems to be unaware of any difficulties in his own sexuality and seems quite happily heterosexual.

John is using the defence mechanism of denial here. Some people repeat the pattern of being attracted to unavailable or inappropriate 'love objects' again and again.

Case example 8: Short term relationships

> Kirsten is an accounts executive with a large marketing firm. She works long hours, and has a hectic work and social life. Just as a new partner wants to get to know her better, she finds a work crisis to keep them at bay. She says she's too busy for a relationship and that she prefers to 'keep things simple'.

Margolies *et al.* 1987: 232 describe short term relationships as requiring 'less of a commitment to one's [lesbianism]. Living with a lover involves greater social risks and stigmas than having a casual "dating" type relationship.' Whilst it is undoubtedly true that living with a partner involves a greater visibility and therefore potentially more risk of discrimination, I believe Margolies and her colleagues unwittingly fall into a heterosexist trap here, when they imply that co-habitation is a criteria for commitment and that longevity is a more important measure for relationships than their *quality*. Carl (1990) supports this view when he questions the assumptions that coupling and longevity are best. See Simon's discussion of different relational forms in Chapter 6.

Margolies *et al.* (1987) also note that internalized homophobia incorporates the two fears, erotophobia (fear of one's own sexuality) and xenophobia (discomfort with strangeness). The xenophobia can be seen as resulting from fear of parental and social rejection due to one's differentness from expectations. In this way internalized homophobia reveals the struggle of the ego between the superego's rules and the desires of the id. The therapist's task is to help the client make sense of this struggle and find their own equilibrium.

Covert internalized homophobia also operates at a community level. This can lead to some lesbians and gay men holding themselves to a higher than normal standard of conduct and as a result, being unusually critical toward those who do not meet their unrealistic expectations. This contributes to infighting within the lesbian and gay communities and an inclination to enforce morally absolute standards of conduct and political belief. Community debates about political questions, bisexuality, sexual values and ethics frequently take on a morally absolute tone: 'if we find the correct answers to the questions then, perhaps, we will be good enough' (Gonsiorek 1988: 118).

Conclusions

- This chapter has explored the concepts of homophobia and heterosexism. We have seen how society operates to institutionalize prejudice against lesbian, gay and bisexual people and the effect this can have on mental health.
- We have defined heterosexism as institutionalized structures built on belief in the superiority of heterosexuality over alternative identities, and biphobia as prejudice against bisexuals.
- Allport's distinctions between prejudice and discrimination have been set alongside Herek's list of some reasons for maintenance of prejudice.
- Societal homophobia oppresses people from sexual minorities in complex ways through its institutions, including education, work and training, and through its cultural systems – for example, in sports and entertainment – where different sexualities are denied or denigrated.

- In the mental health professions, homophobic and heterosexist bias is evident and must be guarded against in therapy and counselling training, in supervision, consultation and clinical practice. Chapter 2 offered models for training and retraining in affirmative, anti-discriminatory ways.
- Therapists may be presumed heterosexist or become the object of client projections and negative transference, and some clients (and even some supervisees) will self-censor as a result. Where therapists demonstrate willingness to work through their own biases and openness to different experience as well as knowledge of subcultural issues, their heterosexuality has not been experienced as a barrier by their clients or trainees.
- It is impossible for lesbians and gay men *not* to have internalized some negative messages about their sexuality from being raised in this society. Therapists need to be trained, informed and sensitive in assisting clients' healing and restructuring.
- A range of clinical manifestations of internalized oppression have been described, including rationalization, denial, projection, introjection and identification with the aggressor. The therapist's task is to help clients make sense of the conflicts between a rule-bound superego and erotophobia to achieve greater ego stability.

4 | DOMINIC DAVIES

Working with people coming out

This chapter defines and explores the phenomenon known as 'coming out' and why it has become identified as a central part of the development of lesbian and gay identity. It also presents some of the established models of coming out and briefly examines the process in relation to people of colour, people with disabilities, and the implications for people with a bisexual orientation. It explores some of the blocks to coming out and illustrates the process with clinical examples where appropriate.

First it is necessary to define what is meant by 'coming out' and then to explore why coming out is crucial to the development of a healthy identity for lesbians, gay men and bisexuals:

> Coming out involves a complex process of intra- and interpersonal transformations, often beginning in adolescence and extending well into adulthood which lead to, accompany and follow the events associated with acknowledgement of one's sexual orientation.
>
> Hanley-Hackenbruck (1989: 21)

Coming out, as defined by Cohen and Stein (1986: 32),

> refers to a complicated developmental process which involves, at a psychological level, a person's awareness and acknowledgement of homosexual thoughts and feelings. For some persons, coming out ultimately leads to public identification as a gay man or lesbian. Various factors will affect the relative positive or negative meaning the individual places on the identity which emerges as a result of the coming out process.

Why is coming out so important?

Erikson (1946) has shown that an individual needs to accomplish several developmental tasks as they move through his eight stages. Identity development involves the integration of one's sexuality; this is crucial to the well-being of a healthy adult. However, Erikson demonstrates that identity formation is a complex interactive process between the individual and society. Since the development of a lesbian or gay identity differs significantly from that of a heterosexual identity and the norms of British society remain largely anti-gay, then the development of gay men and lesbians must mean the integration of a stigmatized aspect of identity. This stigmatization, described in detail in the previous chapter, has become known as homophobia.

There have been a number of psychological models of coming out developed over the last two decades (Grace 1977; de Monteflores and Schultz 1978; Kimmel 1978; Cass 1979; Troiden 1979; Woodman and Lenna 1980; Coleman 1981/82; McDonald 1982; Minton and McDonald 1983/84). In this chapter three quite different models are explored: Cass, Coleman and Woodman and Lenna. They can be seen as complementary, though aspects of them could be viewed as conflicting. As Chapter 1 argued, there are no clear and definitive 'causes' for a lesbian or gay orientation, and so the process of acknowledging and coming to terms with that orientation is also open to debate. These three models are given to help therapists and clients locate phases of development in at least one.

One of the major difficulties in presenting these models is that they seem to be based on the assumption that one is either heterosexual *or* gay. This fallacy was countered in the first chapter. However it is a fundamental flaw in the work of many therapists and researchers that they have made this assumption. It can therefore be confusing for the therapist and indeed sometimes for the client, whether the person has a 'genuine' bisexual orientation or there are defence mechanisms being utilized (resistance to accepting their homosexuality). Since sexual orientation is known to change in many people over time, then perhaps *sometimes* there is both resistance to identifying as someone who has same sex relationships *and* a bisexual orientation – at one time a rationalization, a denial of their homosexuality, and at another, a genuine bisexual orientation.

It is important that the models should not be seen as describing a linear progressive continuum. People usually do not simply pass sequentially from one stage to another (McDonald 1982), and a client may be working on the developmental tasks of several stages simultaneously. All such psychological models should only be seen as descriptive of where someone is now and cannot be used in a predictive way. However, they do offer a useful theoretical construct to help the client and therapist make sense of what has been observed or experienced. It is proposed that a person needs to have worked through each of the stages described for them to be fully integrated in their sexual identity, although this should not imply that their identity will necessarily be fixed.

The process of coming out is also heavily influenced by a number of significant variables: gender, race or ethnic group, locale (especially urban vs rural), the extent of sexual variation, the values and attitudes of society at the time, individual variation (including the individual's own psychological make-up, family circumstances, etc.), and physical ability or sensory impairment. It seems appropriate to explore some of these issues in greater depth.

Gender

Because of the differences in socialization for men and women within our society, the process of coming out for each gender will be somewhat different. Lesbians are first socialized into female roles and their responses to coming out are shaped by this role training (Groves and Ventura 1983). Some of the significant differences here are that:

1 Most men become sexually active with male partners before suspecting they may be gay (Weinberg 1978). Most women have few or no sexual experiences with other women prior to suspecting their lesbianism (Ventura 1983).
2 Gay men usually become involved in a committed relationship after accepting their gayness (Troiden 1979), whereas many women become involved in a relationship prior to accepting themselves as lesbians (Cronin 1974; Ventura 1983).
3 There is also a difference in the age at which lesbians and gay men first became aware of their homosexual feelings. Jay and Young (1979) report the median age for awareness in their sample for females was 18 years old and for males 13–14 years.
4 Bell and Weinberg (1978) have shown that over 90 per cent of lesbians have a history of sexual involvement with men, many having been married: this is not usual for gay men.

Race

Almost all minority ethnic groups have moral objections, usually on religious grounds, to homosexuality. A member of a minority ethnic group has undoubtedly been exposed to racial prejudice. However, racial identity is supported and reinforced, at least by their family. It can be extremely difficult, therefore, if someone has a growing realization of a different sexual orientation, because this is likely to meet with disapproval and possibly rejection by their family and community. This is compounded by the fact of racial prejudice from the majority white community. A recent example of this was the case of the black British footballer, Justin Fashanu, who came out as gay in October 1990. A major black community newspaper *The Voice* gave headline coverage to the initial rejection of Justin by his brother, and several other anti-gay articles were featured.

Whilst it is still difficult for white lesbians and gay men to see positive role models of 'competent' out lesbians and gay men, there are virtually no ethnic minority public figures who are openly gay. This contributes to low self-esteem and feelings of isolation experienced by many lesbians and gay men from ethnic minorities.

Locale

There are obvious advantages to living in a large city. It is highly likely that there will be 'visible' lesbians and gay men, and in many cities there are social groups and possibly even a local gay switchboard or lesbian line. The lesbian or gay man living in a rural setting may well experience profound isolation, often believing that they are the only one in their town or village (see Chapter 5). This is statistically unlikely but one of the problems of growing up gay in our society is access to accurate information; someone living in a rural community is unlikely to have access to gay newspapers, literature, social groups and so on. Their only encounter with gay issues may be occasional television or radio programmes and, if they are male, writing on the public toilet walls – hardly a positive view of lesbian and gay life! Where attitudes may be negative and where fears of reprisals may be stronger, the coming out process is typically prolonged or foreclosed entirely out of fear, lack of knowledge or support and dependence upon a non-accepting environment.

Extent of sexual variation

As stated earlier, most researchers and clinicians view sexual orientation as a dichotomy: one is either heterosexual or homosexual. For someone coming out as bisexual, or who has a substantial hetero- or homosexual component, their process may be affected by the absence of much in the way of organized support systems and bi-positive organizations. Many lesbians and gay men are '*biphobic*' (see Chapter 3) just as many heterosexuals are homophobic. It may be easier for someone who is bisexual to come out as lesbian or gay first, since there are more support organizations and community resources to help affirm this identity. However, if that person subsequently wants to come out as bisexual, they risk being isolated by their existing gay support systems.

For the bisexual person moving from a heterosexual identity there is a double coming out with the tasks of acknowledging same sex feelings and attractions as well as establishing a bisexual identity. For the lesbian or gay man, who may have fought over many years to establish this identity, there is the threat of disruption to it if they are to acknowledge and act on their bisexual feelings.

In discussing models of coming out here we have taken gay and lesbian to include bisexuals.

Prevailing attitudes and values

Arguably the best time to come out in Britain was in the late 1970s and early 1980s, especially if one lived in London. This was the period of the Gay Liberation Front (GLF) and the pre-AIDS era. The moral backlash led by the tabloid press against gay men as a result of the AIDS epidemic has made it difficult to come out as lesbian or gay in the late 1980s and 1990s.

The local climate concerning attitudes and values will, axiomatically, have a bearing on the person's intrapsychic processes regarding the 'appropriateness' of their coming out, as well as society's reaction to their disclosure. This is why it is unrealistic for therapists to imagine they can work with clients' issues of sexual identity without cognizance of wider social, cultural and political contexts.

Individual variation

There are many other factors which can affect the coming out process. Hanley-Hackenbruck (1989: 25) reminds us that, as with any developmental process:

> Individual variables lead to the widest variation in the process not only in timing and sequences but also progression through the stages and the ease or difficulties encountered with the tasks involved in each stage. The individual nuances of this identity process are innumerable and are related to variables such as personality and characterological make-up, age at first awareness of difference, overall psychological functioning, family rigidity (especially regarding sexuality), religious upbringing and negative or traumatic experiences involving sexual orientation.

The therapist needs to be aware of these differences and how they can contribute to the process.

Physical and sensory impairment

This will also affect the way in which someone comes out as lesbian or gay. People with disabilities will have many obstacles to their coming out.

Consider the situation of a severely disabled wheelchair user. She may know she is lesbian, but also be highly dependent on able-bodied carers to take her to places (access to the majority of pubs and clubs involves stairs; many are underground or on the first floor of a building), and to do her shopping. The lesbian and gay press may be unavailable outside of gay venues, radical and alternative book shops or the more liberal libraries. One of the most critical issues is the potential homophobia of the carers. Many disabled people are cared for by their parents and others are in the fortunate position, like some students in higher education, of having community service volunteers. It may still be extremely difficult for the person to come out to, and rely on the support of, helpers who may have difficulties with their own sexuality.

Access to helplines is usually limited to people who are able to use the telephone – this may exclude those with speech and hearing difficulties. Many helplines have not yet availed themselves of the technology now available to deaf people by installing text phones. These relatively cheap pieces of equipment enable communication with deaf people by way of ordinary phone lines.

Access to written information, textbooks (numerous gay people mention having scoured the libraries for information about homosexuality), and lesbian and gay literature (which can help to affirm and develop positive self-esteem), are all likely to be denied people with visual difficulties. Incidentally, the *Pink Paper* (see Appendix 2) *is* available on tape.

Quality of therapy

How a client progresses through the coming out process will also depend on how they experience their therapist. There will be both transference and reality-based reactions of clients to the therapist as well as the counter-transference reactions of the therapist to take account of. This is one of the reasons for high quality supervision or consultation by someone who is experienced in working with lesbians and gay men, so that one can be alert to these issues and respond appropriately.

The Woodman and Lenna model

Woodman and Lenna (1980) offer the following model, which I would define as primarily an intrapsychic one since it focuses on the individual's internal world and psychological processes. This is a four stage model, not dissimilar to Kübler-Ross's stages of loss and bereavement (Kübler-Ross 1969). The stages are: denial, identity confusion, bargaining and depression. Woodman and Lenna do not assume that satisfactory resolution of lesbian or gay identity ends in depression, but rather, that resolution of depression results in a healthy integration of their orientation.

Denial

In this phase the client may engage in homosexual activities but would not perceive their feelings or behaviour as gay. They may present to the counsellor for help with something totally unrelated to their sexual orientation.

Case example 1

Alec (19) consulted me at a student counselling service with panic attacks and insomnia. Things had got so much worse for him since coming to university. It seemed difficult for him to identify what it was that was troubling him and only after some weeks of developing a trusting relationship did he feel safe enough to bring some of his dreams. At first the references to homoerotic content were obscure, but eventually he was able to share his feelings of attraction to some of the other men in his hall. As he came to understand and accept his homosexual feelings, so his panic attacks subsided and he was able to resume a normal sleep pattern.

It is also usual to see the operation of ego defence mechanisms in order to manage the feelings or behaviours that cannot be denied – repression, rationalization or projection may be in evidence. Alec provides an example of repression in action. The client who utilizes rationalization can find many reasons to justify their behaviour 'just this time'.

Case example 2

Brian was a keen sportsman, an active member of the Rugby XV and the stereotypical 'lad about town'. He would regularly date extremely attractive women, whom he would 'wear' on his arm at the nightclub and disco, like a bracelet. He found it difficult to express emotional intimacy with his girlfriends and sex was functional and devoid of any tenderness. Increasingly he sought out the company of gay men in pubs, usually when drunk, and would allow himself to be picked up and go home with these men for sex. The following day, he would claim not to remember too much of the night before, because of being so drunk. Later he rationalized that sex was more easily available and less complicated from gay men than from women and so if he felt sexually frustrated he would go directly to gay pubs and clubs.

A more subtle example of denial is through the defences of sublimation and suppression.

Case example 3

Colin was a married computer programmer. He was extremely successful at work, not least because he spent 12 to 18 hours a day there.

His marriage was suffering and he was under stress. One way in which he sought to relieve the stress was through the use of heterosexual pornography. He would 'consume' large quantities of hardcore pornography (the 'live action' type) and it emerged during therapy that the focus of his attention was the men. It appeared that by using the pornography he could believe he was a 'normal' heterosexual man, enjoying looking at other women. In fact, he was being excited by the idea of performing oral sex on a man, or watching other men performing vaginal and anal intercourse on women. For him this was sex without any responsibility to himself or his partner. No one knew what was going on inside his head and he did not need to confront the bisexual or homosexual side of himself.

Identity confusion

In this stage, clients suspect they may be gay, but are usually unhappy about it. They see the therapist as a resource for helping them understand their sexual orientation better and helping them handle the conflict.

Case example 4

Dawn worked as a bank clerk and had for some time realized her attraction to other women. At her counsellor's suggestion she plucked up courage to telephone the local lesbian line. She was met by one of the women volunteers and they went to a lesbian-run pub. In the course of the evening Dawn was introduced to a number of other lesbians, all of whom had come to a political understanding of their lesbianism through feminism. Dawn presented at her next counselling session feeling depressed and even more isolated. 'Those women were just like men. They were all so aggressive. If that's what being a lesbian means then I'm clearly not lesbian.' Dawn felt hurt and alienated by the other women, who had a greater awareness of the oppression of women and had found strength in their identities as women by not conforming to what heterosexual men would want of them (to be feminine, gentle and submissive). However, Dawn at that stage needed to find women who looked like her and who held similar views to hers. She was also angry at her counsellor for not helping her to make contact with lesbians like her.

Thus it is important that therapists are aware of how lesbian and gay agencies work and what the local lesbian and gay social scene offers. This will help the therapist prepare the client for the experience of meeting others and maybe anticipate the possibility of the above scenario.

A further, fairly common example of the projection of anger on to other gays is anger at lesbian and gay activists who are 'blatant' about their sexuality, and in particular, anger projected towards camp or 'effeminate' gay men 'giving the rest of us a bad name'.

Case example 5
Anger may also be projected on to the therapist. If the client considers some aspect of homosexuality negatively and the therapist is open to it, then the therapist may be viewed negatively.

> Elaine came from a strongly religious family. She had been brought up believing that homosexuality was a mortal sin. When she presented to her therapist, and the therapist was quite accepting of her homosexual thoughts and feelings, even encouraging Elaine to consider meeting other young lesbians, she became quite aggressive. She was shocked and angry that the therapist was not behaving like she suspected her parents would.

Alternatively, clients may be well aware of the damage done by therapists who have attempted to 'cure' lesbians and gay men, and possibly even to themselves previously, and be seeking the present therapy only as a last resort. They may therefore be hostile and the therapist will need to help the client express anger about this without becoming defensive.

Clients may also feel that in order to be lesbian or gay, they need to conform to heterosexist stereotypes of lesbians and gay men. For example, women may feel they need to develop a 'butch' appearance, wear their hair short and drink pints; gay men that they should become 'effeminate' and 'queeny'. Partly due to the lack of visibility of the diversity of lesbians and gay men in society, many people, especially young people, feel that they need to conform to these stereotypes to identify, or to be accepted, as lesbian or gay.

Bargaining

At this point the client, overwhelmed by the implications of their gayness, wants to become heterosexual, or to revert to their former lifestyle and identity. The client may see the therapist as an external superego and want them to change reality. It is also likely to be a time when family or spouses may suggest someone enters therapy in order to help them become 'more heterosexual'.

The therapist needs to be aware that there is no basis for a 'cure' (Tripp 1975) and that contracting to work on one is unethical (see Chapter 2 for a detailed discussion). However, the therapist must also be aware that the client may displace anger onto the therapist when told this. A helpful stance is to affirm the client in their ability to take control over their own behaviour and to be clear about what the therapist *can* offer. The client should not be made to feel guilty for wanting to try other options, or for leaving therapy for a while. A non-defensive, professional stance of empathic concern can help the client refocus anger and explore its real source, i.e. those who seek to control the clients' behaviour.

Religious issues may also surface during this phase. 'Can I believe my homosexuality is right with God, even if those in my church disagree?' There is currently some theological support for a lesbian and gay lifestyle and referral to one of the support agencies can be most useful (see Chapter 13 and Appendix 2 for further information).

Depression

When clients have been unsuccessful in finding workable coping mechanisms they may enter this phase. The client is well aware of their gay orientation and rather than project anger on to others, they now direct anger and feelings of guilt at themselves.

One of the major problems for the client in coming to terms with their gay orientation is the real or presumed loss of support from family and friends. Self-esteem is reinforced through our interaction with significant others. To have them withdraw their love and support and not to be in the position of having alternative sources of support is extremely threatening. Furthermore, the client may devalue other lesbians and gay men and so not experience them as positive role models.

The levels of depression seen in clients in this phase can be severe. Suicidal ideation is common as is suicidal and self-destructive behaviour. In a survey conducted for the London Lesbian and Gay Teenage Group, 20 per cent of respondents under 21 years old reported attempting suicide because they were lesbian or gay (Trenchard and Warren 1984). A similar figure has been reported elsewhere (Hetrick and Martin 1987). The therapist needs to be alert to this and be comfortable in asking about suicidal thoughts and feelings. Referral to medical and psychiatric services may need to be considered. An active, empathic concern, accompanied by acceptance of the clients' negative and hopeless feelings, in which the therapist holds the hope, is crucial. It is also important for the therapist to be aware of the possibility of rage and anger being turned inward and clients' wanting to kill themselves to punish others for their gayness, or to end the pain of their 'existence' as lesbian or gay.

The client needs to be able to express their deepest feelings of guilt and anger which are the underlying dynamics for the depression. This may be difficult for the client working with an openly lesbian or gay therapist, since there will be transference and reality-based fears involved. In facilitating expression of painful feelings, the therapist should also help the client identify good things about being lesbian or gay. It must be emphasized that successful resolution of the depression will be essential to identity integration.

Woodman and Lenna pay little attention to what acceptance of a same sex orientation is like. It will be considerably more than the absence of depression! Their model implies that a fully integrated person, having passed through the four phases, will be free of any defensive resistance to their homosexuality. The model which follows represents more of the diverse intrapsychic and interpersonal processes a person is likely to experience in coming to terms with a sexual orientation differing from cultural expectations.

The Cass model

The second model can be seen as an *interactionist* one and was developed by the Australian psychologist, Vivienne Cass (1979). It is based on the two assumptions that we acquire our sexual identities through a developmental process and that stability and change in our behaviour lies in the interaction that occurs between ourselves and society. The framework for the theory is one of interpersonal congruence (Secord and Backman 1961, 1964a, 1974) between the person's *'self'*, their *behaviour* and how these two factors might be perceived by the *outside world*. A complex interaction exists between these three elements and each needs to be in harmony with the other. When this harmony is disturbed the person needs to find another way of reaching a state of equilibrium.

Cass describes an interactionist framework where the individual has the opportunity to progress through up to six stages of identity development, or may stop at any time along the way, until incongruence causes them to move on again. Growth occurs when the individual attempts to resolve the inconsistency between their perception of self and others at both a cognitive and affective level. The six stages are: identity confusion; identity comparison; identity tolerance; identity acceptance; identity pride and identity synthesis.

Identity confusion

Before this stage an individual would normally view themselves as heterosexual, since that is the way society expects everyone to be and those who are have had no need to examine the presumption of heterosexuality. The situation is not the same for someone who becomes conscious of a sense of difference. This stage begins, therefore, with an individual becoming aware that homosexuality has a relevance to themselves (either through having participated in some kind of homosexual behaviour, or the awareness of thoughts, emotions or physiological responses to same sex stimuli). The thought, which may not be verbalized, is that 'my behaviour may be labelled lesbian or gay'. This can lead to feelings of alienation from society.

Someone in this situation could react in a number of ways. She might like the idea of being seen as lesbian and so begin to actively question her orientation by searching out lesbian related books, listening to lesbian identified conversations and so on. She might see her behaviour as lesbian, but feel very uncomfortable about this and so stop any behaviour that might be labelled as lesbian, avoid and ignore any references to homosexuality or deny any personal relevance. The success of this strategy may be enhanced by adopting a strong anti-homosexual stance (the 'moral crusader') or becoming asexual, or throwing herself with a vengeance back into a heterosexual identity – perhaps by marrying.

Whether she is able to achieve this avoidance will, Cass suggests, depend on her ability to withdraw from potentially provocative situations. It may be easier to give up going to dyke bars, but harder to stop dreaming about sex with Sigourney Weaver, or feeling aroused when someone she has a crush on enters the room. It will also depend on her ability to utilize the defence mechanism known as 'denial' and her ability to maintain an image of asexuality or heterosexuality (e.g. there may be family pressure on her to get married and settle down).

The third approach to resolving the incongruities of this stage is to see her behaviour as wrong and her identity as non-gay. This might be the case if she were engaged in sexual relationships whilst in a single sex environment like a girl's boarding school or women's prison. Alternatively, she may come to view strong emotional feelings for another woman as acceptable, but genital contact would not be. The opposite may be true for a man adopting this position, it may be all right to fool around sexually with another man, but not to kiss or show any affection. The 'I'm not gay because I'm not effeminate' scenario would also apply in this situation. They would view their behaviour not as homosexual, but as an 'experiment' or, in the case of some rent boys, as a way of earning some money or else a way in which they were 'taken advantage' of.

Identity comparison

The task of this phase is to resolve the dilemma of 'Who am I?' and to cope with the social alienation that arises following acceptance that one may be homosexual. The individual knows that she's attracted to, and feels sexually aroused by, other women but is acutely aware that this is not how other people feel. She feels alienated from society, her family and possibly from her friends too. As she comes to accept that she isn't heterosexual, she will also be questioning her previously held ideals, values and expectations for the future. She may not be about to get married, set up home and have children, with a loving family and in-laws who support her and share in the child care. In addition to questioning all these guidelines for behaviours and values, she is aware that they have not yet been replaced by others and will now have the task of developing a personally relevant value system and her own meanings for life.

The alienation she feels may lead her to seek contact with other lesbian and gay people. If she feels very uncomfortable about her 'differentness', she may seek therapy, with the goal of 'I don't want to be different'. The therapist, as has been seen in the first chapters of this book, will know it is futile to focus on her homosexuality as something that needs to be changed; rather, it is working through her feelings of difference and dealing with the loss of familiar structures that are the tasks of therapy.

There are four approaches open to the individual who wishes to reduce feelings of alienation in this stage. The first is to feel positively about differentness, in terms of the new identity and sexual behaviour. There are generally three groups of people who feel good about the adoption of a gay identity:

1 The individual who has always felt different to others by having had what were later labelled as homosexual feelings, thoughts or behaviour. Having a label for herself and realizing that there are others who feel this way helps her feel she belongs somewhere, a sort of 'coming home'.
2 The individual who has felt different all of her life on the basis of her non-conformity to the stereotypical gender role (e.g. someone who never saw why she should get married and have children).
3 The individual who finds being 'different' exciting and out of the ordinary. She sees her sexual identity as another way in which she can be different to 'normal' people, more special perhaps.

Whilst the individual may well be saying to herself, 'I now don't care what others think of me', they are still likely to be presenting an image of heterosexuality which will, of course, protect them from experiencing negative views of lesbians and gay men. This 'passing' is easy because it means just following old patterns of behaviour. However, there may be difficulties in this. Only if the person can use the following strategies will passing work for them:

- avoiding threatening situations (e.g. the Christmas party where one is expected to take along a partner of the other sex);
- controlling personal information (e.g. not talking about what one did at the weekend and dressing carefully, so as not to give anyone the impression one might be lesbian or gay);
- deliberately cultivating an image of heterosexuality or asexuality; and
- 'role distancing' – appearing detached from the lesbian or gay situation (e.g. not supporting lesbian or gay colleagues at work for fear of guilt by association and not voicing objections to anti-gay abuse).

When passing is undetected then incongruence is reduced, but not eliminated. One can imagine the stress of trying to lead this hidden lifestyle.

This has been described as being like a spy in an enemy occupied country (Ratigan 1991).

The second approach occurs when an individual accepts their homosexual behaviour, but doesn't like the idea of a homosexual self-identity. She can achieve this by adopting the following strategies:

1 *Special case strategy*: She sees herself as lesbian only in relation to her current partner. 'If it weren't for Janet, I'd be married with kids by now.'
2 *Ambisexual strategy*: The individual perceives herself as capable of having both heterosexual and same sex relationships. She need not actually have a heterosexual relationship, but just feel she could if she wanted to. 'Freud said everyone is bisexual' and pointing out famous bisexuals are common strategies for someone in this position.
3 *Temporary identity strategy*: 'I'm only gay at the moment. I'll probably end up getting married later.'
4 *Personal innocence strategy*: This strategy may be adopted by someone who, whilst accepting they are lesbian or gay, view their sexuality very negatively. 'I was born this way. It's not my fault', seeing themselves as victims of misfortune. The person who adopts this line is likely to develop a negative identity characterized by self-hate.

The third approach to handling the incongruence in this stage is when the person accepts their homosexual identity but, because of strong feelings of social alienation, is scared to translate this desire into behaviour. This is particularly likely to be the case where the person fears rejection by family, peers or their church. It is here that the person may be saying, 'I may be gay but it is wrong for me to practise.' Help from doctors, therapists or religious leaders may be sought to help reduce homosexual desires.

The fourth approach is when the person sees gay identity and gay behaviours as undesirable and wants to change both. They may try to achieve this by avoiding anything to do with homosexuality or by devaluing it. It is difficult for this strategy to be successful for long without serious consequences to self-esteem. The individual is left with such a profound sense of self-hatred that, should their strategy fail, they could become suicidal.

Identity tolerance

By the end of the previous stage, assuming that the person has not foreclosed their sexual identity, they are likely to have a greater commitment to a gay identity and be saying 'I am probably lesbian/gay/bisexual.' The individual will be spending increasing time seeking contact with other lesbians, gay men or bisexuals in order to compensate for feelings of alienation from heterosexual society. The way this is approached though is more akin to 'something has to be done' rather than a keen embracing of the wish to socialize. The individual tolerates, rather than accepts, their identity. They feel increasingly detached from heterosexual others and begin to choose very carefully who they socialize with.

With regard to their contact with others, it is the *quality* of contact which is important at this time. Should they have positive encounters then they are likely to progress on to the next stage. However, many factors can contribute to a negative experience: shyness, poor social skills, low self-esteem, fear of exposure, and internalized homophobia. Whilst some people might find a night out at a disco an exciting thing, for others it may be a very boring or even frightening experience. 'If discos (one night stands, or whatever) are what being gay is all about then I do not want to be gay.' The individual may then reduce contact or tell themselves, 'I am probably lesbian/gay but I don't like it.' It is likely that someone adopting this position will continue, albeit in a reduced way, to meet other lesbian or gay people. Or they may adopt a self-hating position – 'I don't want to be homosexual' – and inhibit homosexual behaviour and contact entirely.

Mixing within the subculture offers much that is positive. It affords opportunities, for example, to meet a partner. Isay (1989) believes that for some, 'falling in love is the only experience that can overcome the resistance and denial produced by years of alienation and self-disgust.' The subculture can additionally provide positive role models who present gayness as acceptable, the opportunity to feel more at ease in the new identity through socialization, and a ready made support group. Aspects of these issues, which may be perceived or experienced as negative, might include the demand for a greater commitment to a gay identity and the possible disclosure of their gayness by people they meet to others outside the gay communities.

However, as before, the individual can go one of two ways at this time. Some experience their contacts with other gay people as desirable and affirming and move on to the next stage. Others, accepting their need for same sex contact and behaviour, will not wish for a lesbian or gay *identity*. This group will continue to rationalize their behaviour in ways outlined previously (special case, ambisexual, temporary identity and personal innocence). If identity foreclosure does not occur, then by the end of this stage the person will be able to accept that they are lesbian, gay or bisexual.

Identity acceptance

Due to greater socialization into the subculture, the individual now develops supportive friendships. They will view other gay people positively and give them at least equal significance in their life. Whether they progress through the remaining two stages will depend upon the influence of those they mix with.

Some people hold the view that it is important to have both a personal and a public identity as lesbian or gay. Others believe that it is fine to be gay in private and amongst chosen heterosexual friends, but not something one should 'display' to the rest of society, by the wearing of gay identified badges, for example, or taking part in social or political action, marches and so on.

This philosophy of 'fitting in' concurs with the individuals' previous behaviour of 'passing'. To this strategy may now be added limited contact with other lesbians and gays and selective disclosure, which may function to protect the individual's 'secret'. They may reduce contact with people who might threaten to disturb their comfort with the newly accepted identity (i.e. families, homophobic friends). Living arrangements and jobs may be changed in order to protect them from experiencing incongruence between themselves and others' negative views. For many this is a satisfactory way to live their lives.

Others decide that 'passing' is now unacceptable, find that the incongruence (personal dishonesty) is heightened and move on to the next stage.

Identity pride

It is at this point that the individual feels that their identity is totally acceptable and that society's rejection of them is wrong. They therefore develop strategies to split society into the 'baddies', who are discredited and devalued (heterosexuals), and the 'goodies' who are 'my people'. The individual throws themselves into the gay communities, consuming all things gay: literature, theatre, dance etc. Other lesbian and gay people are the only source of real friendship and become the 'significant others'. There is a strong sense of pride in one's identity; 'Glad to be Gay', the anthem of the 1970s, would be particularly relevant for people in this stage.

Alongside this pride are feelings of anger that heterosexual society has alienated them and devalues the same sex love and affection that is central to their identity. This combination of anger and pride creates an 'activist'. The individual is now largely unconcerned with how they are perceived by heterosexuals and free to disclose whenever they feel like it. This is helpful in that it increases the congruence between the private and the public identities.

Inevitably, there will be occasions where it is felt prudent not to disclose (e.g. where it might cost them their job, or result in physical danger); however, it may be that concealing one's identity is seen as a compromise here.

Identity synthesis

The individual enters this stage when the 'them and us' strategy is no longer useful or true. With increased contact with supportive heterosexuals, the person can begin to realize that many heterosexuals are not hostile and do not support the alienation of heterosexism.

This positive contact helps the individual to see considerable similarities between themselves and their heterosexual friends and acknowledge some dissimilarities between themselves and some lesbian and gay people. Instead of seeing themselves primarily as a lesbian or a gay man, they now view their sexuality as part of their total identity. No matter how well integrated someone is, there will still be a power difference between them and heterosexuals which will make total integration impossible, at least for the foreseeable future.

The Coleman model

The third model was developed by Eli Coleman (1981/82), who proposes a five stage model which describes many of the factors seen in individuals coming out. His stages are: pre-coming out, coming out, exploration, first relationships and identity integration.

Pre-coming out

We do not know what causes someone to be attracted to another of the same sex and there has been much research into this (see Chapter 1). However, Coleman adopts the view, put forward by Money and Ehrhardt (1972), that gender and sex-role identities are formed by 3 years of age. Money and Ehrhardt believe that sexual object choice is an integral component of gender identity and, therefore, that the origins of sexuality are determined during the period of late infancy and early childhood. Coleman points out that whilst this needs further substantiation, it seems an idea worthy of serious consideration. If we assume that our sexual identities are formed by that age, then it is clearly possible that on a conscious or preconscious level the parents and the child know that the child is in some way 'different'. It is during these early years that the child acquires family values and attitudes, to (homo)sexuality amongst other things. The child may be aware of their difference and know that they may be rejected and ridiculed should they make it explicit. They grow up with lowered self-esteem and use a variety of defence mechanisms to protect themselves and their families from the crisis that would erupt if their homosexuality became known.

At the pre-coming out stage many individuals are not consciously aware of same sex feelings and so cannot describe what is wrong. They may communicate their conflict through behavioural problems or psychosomatic illness or suicide attempts. Lesbians and gay men often have an experience of being 'different' many years in advance of being able to label that difference 'lesbian' or 'gay' (Jay and Young 1979).

Coming out

This stage begins with what Plummer (1975) refers to as 'those first conscious and semi-conscious moments in which an individual comes to perceive himself as homosexual'. The developmental task an individual faces in this stage is disclosure to others. The purpose is to receive external validation. Obviously, if the disclosure goes well, the individual will feel a rise in self-esteem and the positive attitude of the other person will help counteract some of the years of negative conditioning. If the disclosure goes badly however, their internalized shame and guilt will be confirmed. It is therefore a critical time and most often helped by having first developed a support network of other lesbians or gay men who accept and affirm the individual as a lesbian or gay person. Dank (1973) found that the frequency of feelings of guilt and loneliness, as well as the need for psychiatric or psychological consultations, decreased as the person spent more time living with their homosexual identity. However, for a secure and positive identity to be formed it is likely to be necessary for the person to take risks such as disclosing to non-gay significant others. The therapist can help the client work on who to tell and how to cope with their reaction. It may be helpful to remind clients that they had difficulties in accepting themselves and held negative views of their gay identity and so it is possible that some of the people they tell might find it difficult to accept at first. However, people who really love the individual will, in time, accept their gayness as a part of their whole identity.

Exploration

This stage involves the process of socialization into lesbian and gay communities. The person has been socialized as a heterosexual and now needs to develop the skills of meeting and socializing with others with similar sexual interests, and to develop self-esteem and self-confidence about their gay aspects (which may be different from their heterosexually acquired skills and attributes). Isay (1989: 61) states: 'Relationships that are mutual and loving, both sexual and non-sexual, are essential to the healthy integration of a homosexual identity, promoting a positive self image.'

Some individuals and society at large view the sexual and social experimentation that accompanies this stage as 'immature, immoral and merely promiscuous' (Coleman 1981/82). However, it is helpful to view this as the experience of a delayed adolescence which can be seen as a 'developmental lag' (Grace 1977), where the lesbian or gay man is living out the adolescence they were unable to have during their teenage years.

First relationships

Eventually the need for intimacy takes over and the person begins to have 'relationships' (as distinct from 'encounters'). These are similar to adolescent relationships and often are characterized by intensity, possessiveness and lack of trust. There is a desperation to make the relationship succeed, yet there are few role models of visible, successful long term relationships to emulate (see Chapter 6).

Many gay men in particular can get stuck in a cycle of exploration and brief but intense relationships. This may be because of an unresolved grief reaction to relationship breakdown.

Identity integration

Finally there is the incorporation of public and private identities into one self. Coleman reminds us that this is a lifelong process. Relationships are now characterized by openness, non-possessiveness, mutual trust and freedom.

Coleman appears to ignore the intrapsychic ambivalence that most lesbians and gay men go through in coming to terms with their sexual orientation. He doesn't identify any of the defence mechanisms that the other two models present, but it is a gay affirmative model. His employment, for example, of the concept of 'developmental lag' throws light where previously gay men have been accused of being only interested in sex and incapable of forming meaningful relationships. The model is also more clearly relevant to gay men. This is the group he conducted his research with, and generalizations to include lesbians or bisexuals may not necessarily be valid.

Conclusions

This chapter has described a number of key features in the coming out process for lesbians and gay men. Many of these will also be experienced by men and women coming out as bisexual, since it is the healthy integration of a stigmatized identity which forms one of the major tasks of coming out, and bisexuality is also a stigmatized identity.

- 'Coming out' is a complex developmental process of intrapsychic and interpersonal transformations extending well into adulthood, with a range of different outcomes, not a once-and-for-all event.
- This process is crucially interrelated to the development of personal and social identity, self-esteem and authentic, satisfying relations with others.

- The models discussed are not linear and sequential, but describe interdependent developmental phases, each having identifiable tasks requiring resolution; they are not to be seen as prescriptive. Clients may be working on several developmental tasks at once.
- The three models given are not regarded as definitive and are flawed in adopting bipolar approaches to the spectrum of human sexuality.

PART II

Working with particular issues

5 | LYNDSEY MOON

Working with single people

Community

When working with lesbian, gay and bisexual people, therapists need to be aware of the diversity within these particular client groups. It is important to consider the meaning of terms such as 'gay community' and worthwhile at this point considering what a lesbian, gay or bisexual lifestyle means to you – disregarding media representations. In effect, lifestyle refers to what we 'do', while community refers to 'where' this takes place. For some people, the way a particular style of life is created depends on the particular community they feel most at home with. For example, some lesbians may want to explore their interests in fetish or leather sex while others (and some from the latter groups!) may want to campaign around their rights to have children. Within these activities they meet others who lead similar 'lifestyles' to their own (e.g. have children, support political groups, etc.) and form communities which allow the individual the time and space to maintain or experiment with their lesbian identity. What needs to be remembered is that, rather than thinking in terms of one 'gay community', we will more accurately think in terms of a whole range of lesbian, gay and bisexual communities, held together by a broad diversity of lifestyles and creating a culture that exists both locally and nationally.

This chapter will explore some of the ways single lesbian, gay and bisexual people choose to lead their lives and the communities they have created in order to maintain these lifestyles. The focus will be on single people who want to meet others, and individual concerns that result from participation within communities, as well as on issues raised for those who live outside major towns or cities, have disabilities or are from minority ethnic communities. Therapists will want to understand some of the problems faced by these groups before considering what we can do to support clients who are dealing with them.

Meeting others

It is important to the vast majority of lesbian, gay and bisexual people that there are places to meet – to become a part of a chosen community of like minded others. This may include political, social or leisure environments amongst others. How an individual can begin and maintain an active part will vary, depending on their needs and desires (which may change over time) and the groups in which they feel accepted. For example, lesbian communities provide women with an opportunity to explore and begin to define their own identity. Many lesbians, through heterosexual socialization, may never have had the opportunity to talk through the gap in perception between how they 'ought' to be (e.g. wife, mother, carer, etc.) and how they choose to be. Some may feel they have to be in a relationship to be an 'acceptable' lesbian – without having acknowledged a past history of heterosexual means, values and attitudes attached not only to their sexuality but also to their gender. When working with this client group it is important to allow the individual to work through negative stereotypes of lesbians and women in order to strengthen their identity and self-esteem.

These communities are there to offer mutual support to lesbian, gay and bisexual people who are either coming out or have been out for some years. They provide an invaluable social structure which is beneficial to the development and maintenance of a positive sexual identity. As Gonsiorek and Rudolph (1991) indicate, involvement with a positive ongoing social support network helps the individual adopt an affirmative lesbian, gay or bisexual identity, as well as a positive relationship between self-esteem and acceptance of self.

Single lesbians, gay men and bisexuals face similar life problems to their heterosexual counterparts in a society which privileges couples and families. However, some concerns are unique to, or complicated by, a lesbian or gay orientation (Elfin Moses 1990). In order to resist the pressures of a society which, in the main, views same sex desires as negative and shameful, *being* lesbian, gay or bisexual through participation in subcultural lifestyles contributes to the development of a self in which one's sexuality is valued. Concerns arising for individuals during this process, however, can include body image, physical appearance and attractiveness, and emotional intimacy.

Body image

Within the variety of communities that exist, lesbians and gay men may feel pressurized by their peer group to look or behave in particular ways. For example, gay men have been exposed constantly to the prevailing images of 'body beautiful'; the young, muscular, Adonis physique that has had currency as a gay male ideal. Such messages can create problems with body image and a distorted view of the self in relation to other men. Within some lesbian communities as well, primarily in major cities, the notion of 'body beautiful' is increasing within more affluent groups who have access to more upmarket bars and clubs and begin to wear the 'designer dyke' labels.

Body image, which is part of our overall self-image, is influenced by the messages, both verbal and non-verbal, others communicate to us. In turn, how a person perceives and integrates these messages is important to the development of body image. Physical appearance is only one aspect of our sense of self – despite the emphasis placed on it in some lesbian and gay magazines, advertising and press. If self-image depends exclusively or primarily on body image then the individual is 'asking for psychological trouble' (Etnyre 1990).

The impact of images of exceptionally well developed, fit and healthy bodies, with certain shapes being highly valued, has received plenty of coverage over the past few years. For lesbians and gay men, although this material may be useful as encouragement towards becoming healthy, problems can occur when the individual develops a relentless drive towards 'body perfection' and notions of physical norms become distorted. Similarities in body image problems between heterosexual women and lesbians found by Brand *et al.* (1992: 86) showed that, due to the process of socialization as women, both lesbians and heterosexual women were more likely to experience dissatisfaction with their bodies, greater concern with their weight, and more frequent dieting than did gay or heterosexual men. As they suggest, 'lesbians may be as restricted by the appearance mandates for women as are heterosexual women.' Therapists need to be aware that what constitutes a desirable lesbian body image may be very different from that aspired to by most heterosexual women, despite similar problems.

Anecdotal evidence suggests many publicly 'out' bisexuals are less affected by traditional lesbian and gay concerns over body image and fashion trends. Some bisexuals are experimenting with a more androgynous appearance as a way of integrating and challenging externally imposed norms about masculine and feminine identities imposed equally by heterosexual and homosexual cultures.

Therapists need to be sure they have challenged negative attitudes and stereotypes often flaunted by media publicity regarding the appearance of lesbians and gay men. There is an increased societal pressure to conform to heterosexual standards of appearance – for lesbians to be more 'feminine' and gay men to be more 'masculine' in order to be accepted. Alan Sinfield's *The Wilde Century* (1994) is a highly informative and challenging discussion of cultural notions of 'masculinity', 'femininity', and 'effeminacy' and their relationship to social and psychological oppression. Women have had a lifetime of being told how to look and, as lesbians are women, it is more than likely that socialization and the media representations take their hold even more resolutely. For men it can mean trying to live up to the 'perfect shape' or to ideals of manly behaviour. Gay men place considerable value on the physical appearance of their partner (Blumstein and Schwartz 1983) and, regardless of their own attractiveness, many will prefer partners more attractive than themselves (Sergios and Cody 1985/86). Therapists need to be aware that, despite this, gay men frequently express greater concern with their own body image and feelings about their bodies than any other group (Etnyre 1990). Findings by Silberstein *et al.* (1989) concluded that a male subculture that emphasizes appearance may heighten the vulnerability of its members to body dissatisfaction and disordered eating.

For the therapist it is important to work towards an assessment with the client of options available by exploring the myths and realities concerning their body. The client can decide what they want to do with their body based on inner convictions and feelings, rather than external pressures and media representations, on the basis of strengthened self-esteem.

Case example 1

> Mark was a computer programmer in his late 20s. He moved to London immediately after university, and began his coming out journey. He was referred for therapy by his GP, who recognized early signs of anorexia nervosa.
>
> Mark had joined a gym on coming to London as a result of seeing so many muscle-toned men. He worked out five times a week and had become extremely conscious about his diet, keeping food intake to the barest minimum.
>
> Through therapy he explored his desire to 'fit in' and belong – a feeling he'd had since childhood. It had become especially painful during his teens and university life. Mark felt by working hard on his body image he would become accepted by other gay men. He realized this sense of belonging was very hollow and a great cost to his self-esteem. He spent so much time at the gym, he had little time and energy left for socializing. When someone did invite him out he found eating and drinking in company too painful and so generally declined.
>
> Mark's therapist helped him explore his shame about his sexuality, and his loneliness. Through bibliotherapy he was directed to some

self-help relationship texts, which improved his dating skills and Mark decided to join a social group for gay professionals.

Emotional intimacy

Emotional intimacy has been defined in behavioural terms as mutual self-disclosure and other kinds of verbal sharing, as declarations of liking or loving the other, and as demonstrations of affection such as hugging and non-genital caressing (Lewis 1978).

For emotional intimacy to occur, individuals need to communicate with each other and this may be dependent on earlier experiences of self-disclosure. Self-disclosure is an important part of emotional intimacy and if this was prevented in earlier experience it seems likely that verbal sharing, hugging and liking or loving others will be adversely affected in the forming of later relationships. Chapter 4 indicated some key issues for lesbian, gay and bisexual people around self-disclosure and readers will find in Chapter 8 discussion of the impact of heterosexism on young people attempting to express their selfhood and develop an identity.

For gay men especially, the barriers to intimacy can be immense on the basis of traditional male role models. Lewis (1978) indicated three of these barriers:

1 *competition:* wealth, status and power differentials affecting levels of trust and openness;
2 *aversion to vulnerability and openness with other men:* hiding of feelings and thoughts, fears, anxieties, depression, and affection;
3 *lack of role models:* cultural lack of examples of acceptable affection between men.

These lead to 'lethal aspects of the male role' – that is, lower self-disclosure, lack of self-insight and empathy, incompetence at loving self and others. This condition has been called 'dispiritation' – morale and immunity to diseases decrease as a result of being unable to live 'up' to the stringent ideals of masculinity (Jourard 1971).

Therapists may find it helpful to recommend a number of self-help 'relationship' texts for single and newly coupled people involved in same sex relationships, in particular Clunis and Green (1988), Tessina (1989), Berzon (1990), Isensee (1990), Sanderson (1990, 1993) and Driggs and Finn (1991). As you can see, these books have emerged in the late 1980s and early 1990s and may be unfamiliar to many clients; see Appendix 3 for further details.

Lewis (1978) proposes a way of working with men around these issues through workshops focusing on communication between men. By increasing emotional intimacy an individual learns to share and care for others as well as opening himself to previously unknown feelings and experiences and can develop satisfying and meaningful relationships.

For women it is often assumed, sometimes incorrectly, that due to their gender they are more likely to be open with each other and communicate affection, caring and nurturance unconditionally. Lesbian and bisexual women clients may feel they are too 'giving' or 'caring' towards others without considering their own needs. Therapy sessions can usefully examine these issues in relation to expected role stereotypes.

Self-disclosure, emotional intimacy, body image and physical appearance are factors all lesbian, gay and bisexual people may be faced with during the development of a satisfying sexual identity. It is clear that these factors are interrelated and occur at both intrapsychic and interpersonal levels. Single people may never have been given the opportunity to explore these issues and it raises important questions for therapists that, when working with lesbians, gay men and bisexuals, they are clear how they understand these issues themselves. The importance of the communities in helping the individual explore their identity on a social level cannot be underestimated.

Rural lesbian and gay male lives

The lesbian and gay male social milieu offers wider opportunities for meeting with others than ever before. One look in lesbian, gay and bisexual newspapers and magazines lists a wide variety of different activities from leisure to business (see Appendix 2). Lesbian and gay culture has expanded over the past few years to incorporate a diversity of interests and this appears to be ever increasing – resulting in an expansion of social contacts and increased lesbian, gay and bisexual visibility. However, therapists need to be aware that this expansion is greater in larger towns and cities. For gay men, and lesbians in particular, living in smaller towns and villages can mean that:

> Homosexist circumstances, lack of affirmative resources, and the intrinsic problems of asserting a non-normative affectional life conspire to encourage lesbian women to become 'invisible' in rural settings even more than in metropolitan areas where social opportunities have always been more available for gay men than for women.
>
> (D'Augelli 1989: 121)

(*Homosexism* in this context equates to the disapproval of homosexuality, and is akin to a definition of sexism as the devaluation of women's sexuality.)

It is more likely lesbians and gay men will remain invisible with regard to their sexuality in rural settings and will have to travel to their nearest town in order to meet others. Bisexuals have even greater difficulties in finding social support and 'community'. Due to economic factors, the opportunity for socializing is likely to be limited. Again, it is probable that there are only pubs and clubs on offer – alternative options will be few and often non-existent in smaller communities. For some single people living in rural areas, 'passing' as heterosexual will be the only answer and any contact with a gay 'scene' or other lesbians and gay men will be avoided. For single gay and bisexual men 'cottaging' may be the only access to a network of other men without a 'scene' life. This can create even more pressure; at home there may be a fear of being 'found out', and at work or with friends there can be a constant monitoring of what to say and how to act. As D'Aguelli (1989: 122) suggests:

> In this way, homophobia truncates personal, social and interpersonal development since significant components of identity are withheld, distorted, or rendered superfluous in daily interactions with others . . . due to a fear that 'somehow' 'someone' will 'find out'.

The therapist needs to take into account the problems presented to single lesbian, gay and bisexual people living in rural areas. It is important that the therapist has awareness of social networks and resources available and can explore with the client their social history – past, present and expected – in order to understand the reasons for isolation. These may include individual and social contexts. Care should be taken when looking at possibilities of disclosure to others and always check with the client whether it would be useful to be part of a social network – individual needs and consequences are of primary importance (D'Aguelli 1989).

When working with single people living outside larger towns and cities, the factors mentioned earlier will require careful exploration relative to the impact of living without the support of a lesbian, gay and bisexual culture.

Race and cross-cultural issues

Research focusing on the experiences of lesbians, gay men and bisexuals has remained largely within the 'safety' of white, middle-class, well-educated groups. This ignores the reality of disadvantage and discrimination experienced by ethnic minority groups. Lesbians, gay men and bisexuals from these communities are faced with the dilemma of finding ways of integrating who they are culturally and racially with their sexual identity. They may be confronted with the task of transforming given stigmatized identities through a gradual process which moves from a rejected and denied self-image to the embracing of an identity that is finally accepted as positive (Espin 1987).

Tremble *et al.* (1989) identified the following issues that lesbians and gay men within racial and ethnic minorities have to deal with:

- particular difficulties in coming out to the family;
- finding a niche in the gay and lesbian community in the face of discrimination;
- difficulties in reconciling sexual orientation with ethnic or racial identity.

We have seen how self-disclosure presents many people with complex issues. For lesbians and gay men of visible minorities, unique stresses are encountered as they are more likely to have 'a foot in each culture without feeling a complete sense of belonging to either' (Tremble et al. 1989: 264). When working with people from ethnic and racial minority groups the therapist needs to understand the impact of specific contextual variables (i.e. culture, class, historical context) on the individual client. We need to take into account that the individual may, through disclosure, lose an important connection with his or her culture. What are the present and future practical and psychological implications of this loss? What alternative support networks exist? What do these mean for the individual in relation to his or her identity? For lesbians in particular, there may need to be discussion around what it means to be disconnected from male centred cultural values and the personal losses faced if she has broken strict cultural norms (Espin 1987). The therapist should keep in mind that there is as much danger in explaining individual differences away as culturally determined as there is in ignoring or rejecting the impact of cultural influences on each individual's choices (Espin 1987).

Those from ethnic and racial minorities are confronted by lesbian and gay communities which are largely Eurocentric in culture and value systems. Participation exposes the person to risk of rejection, exposure to racism and pressure to minimize their own culture. Not only does overt racism exist but the expectation that discrimination is likely to occur in a particular environment can affect attitudes and behaviours as the individual seeks to minimize potential occurrences, e.g. avoiding persons and situations where discrimination could arise (Mays et al. 1993).

Case example 2

Kamlesh is an Asian woman in her early 20s. She is involved in postgraduate studies at university and self-refers for counselling because although she knows she is a lesbian, she is struggling to find a way of integrating her sexual identity with her racial and cultural identity. Kamlesh is also lonely and has few friends who know of her sexuality. She is a fairly shy person and prefers quiet interests. She feels she doesn't fit in on the local gay scene, and she knows no other lesbian or gay Asians.

Kamlesh's parents hold traditional beliefs about arranged marriages and the role of women, although they are also keen for her to receive a good education and have a good career.

> Through therapy Kamlesh developed greater self-confidence in her bicultural identity, and she was able to discuss her sexuality after first getting the support of an older brother. Kamlesh also started to occasionally attend the Bhungra (discos) of Shakti – a support group for Asian lesbian, gay and bisexual people and their friends.

The therapist needs to be sensitive to the needs of the client to explore feelings of anger, frustration, pain and grief as well as issues of confrontation and the internalization of negative messages which the experience of discrimination can bring to the individual and which, in turn, have been found to have a definite impact on psychological well-being (Cromwell 1983).

Bisexuals from ethnic and racial minority groups may on the surface be thought to have an easier time in integrating their sexuality, but racism, biphobia and Eurocentrism in western lesbian, gay and bisexual communities, and heterosexism and homophobia from within their own cultures can mean any expression of their sexual identity is truncated or forbidden, and they may remain isolated.

We must be aware of the multiplicity of discrimination which some clients have experienced and work to understand how our own cultural background influences our responses to the client in any counselling relationship; where there is racial difference, aspects of racism must be assumed to exist (Lago and Thompson 1989).

Disability

> People with physical disabilities and chronic illness live in a world where the values, ideals and goals of the dominant culture are based on 'able bodied assumption' – a world in which physical limitations are seen as the exception, viewed as problematic and judged perjoratively.
>
> (Boden 1992: 159)

Although it is estimated that there are over half a million registered lesbians and gay men with disabilities in Great Britain (and many more who are not registered), their experience is rarely recognized. Single people with disabilities face denial and oppression in terms of both their sexuality and disability. Women with disabilities are additionally affected 'because they fit neither the reproductive nor the sexualised role image of women in our society' (Fine and Asch 1985: 91).

The purpose of this section is to provide the therapist with information when working with lesbian, gay and bisexual people with chronic illness or disabilities, and not in any way to suggest that disability leads to psychological problems. Counselling may be beneficial and supportive for those clients newly diagnosed or when an adjustment to a new level of functioning is required by a progression of symptoms of lifelong disability (Boden 1992).

Disability may be visible or invisible, may be child-onset disability or chronic illness, or occur later in life due to a major change in, or impairment of, bodily appearance or functioning (Elfin Moses 1990). The degree of anxiety that results when impairment occurs later in life will depend on three factors:

1 the amount of change or impairment that occurs and how others react;
2 how much value the individual places on these factors; and
3 how much value the individual places on the body part or function that is altered (Hencker 1979).

As sexual identity develops, the lesbian, gay or bisexual with a disability has to deal with notions of 'difference' – being perceived on several counts as 'different' from the dominant heterosexual, able-bodied society. Therapists working with clients with a disability need both an understanding of the experience of difference and an awareness of the societal context confronting disabled lesbians, gay men and bisexuals as members of minority groups in two important respects (Boden 1992).

Nearly two-thirds of the population will experience some form of disability, either temporary or permanent, by the age of 80. Imagine what it would be like if you found yourself with something as awkward as a broken leg. From personal experience I can tell you how difficult it becomes to move around, to travel on public transport and have to rely on others for basic daily needs. Imagine this becomes a permanent part of everyday life. This simple example shows how life would need to alter – how you would have to adapt and change your routine and style of life to fit in with others. Add to this the experiences of coming out and proclaiming a sexuality that has received hostility, ignorance and prejudice, as discussed in Part I. Try to think of ways you would gain access to the lesbian and gay communities – especially if you live outside of a major town or city – and the picture that begins to emerge is one whereby the majority of people remain both non-supportive and non-responsive, if not hostile, to your needs. Many people fear disability, as they may difference of other sorts, and deny sexuality for people with disabilities. Despite this, lesbians, gay men and bisexuals with disabilities are coming out and proclaiming their sexuality with pride (see Shakespeare *et al.* in press).

Physical access to most of the meeting places for lesbian, gay and bisexual people is severely limited. Many clubs are in basements or upstairs, and even where there is a relatively level access, it is rare indeed to find adapted toilets. Efforts are being made by community groups to hold their meetings in accessible premises, but cruising and socializing with one's peers can be a nightmare.

Any alteration in body image caused by impairment or illness may also raise the level of anxiety and the therapist needs to be able to address this and help the individual to find ways of adapting to new situations and levels of ability. Initially there may be shock and denial and the therapist may help the client to acknowledge what is happening so that he or she may adapt to a new way of life and develop new skills.

We need to consider the wide range of disabilities and the obstacles which create the social and structural disadvantages experienced by people with different abilities. For example, lesbian, gay and bisexual people with learning disabilities will need to know what groups are available and how to make contact with others. They may never have experienced this opportunity and may be surprised to receive support and helpful advice. It will be important to know what specialist services are available for those with visual or hearing impairments and how these groups can find other organizations within the lesbian, gay and bisexual communities. Therapists will also need to examine their own reactions to those with disability considering having children and, where this is physiologically impossible, how they can go about fostering or adoption. These are very real issues for those with disability and can be made more awkward if the therapist gives biased or incorrect information. Disabled lesbians and gay men have as much right to parent children and to receive information as anyone else.

The therapist can be helpful by providing information about organizations which can further support their clients. For example, REGARD campaigns and offers advice and support for disabled lesbian, gay and bisexual people; 'Gemma' provides a befriending and information service for lesbians with or without disabilities and details of groups and organizations are listed in the gay magazines and papers (further details in Appendix 2).

Case example 3

> Mary was a partially deaf women in her mid-30s. She worked for a deaf charity as an administrator. She knew she was attracted to other women, but had no sexual relationships with women since boarding school. She found no difficulty in meeting male partners from within the deaf community, but felt increasingly dissatisfied with only acknowledging 'half' her sexuality.
>
> Mary had experienced isolation and subsequent depression when venturing on to the commercial gay scene of pubs and clubs. Mary's therapist helped her explore her feelings of confusion about her bisexuality which were a result of bipolarized thinking about sexuality. Her therapist was also able to tell her about deaf lesbian, gay and bisexual groups and the monthly magazine for bisexuals, *Bifrost*. Through this she learned of the annual bisexual conference, Bicon. Bicon has a strong equal access policy and provides sign language

interpreters and holds their national gathering in wheelchair accessible premises (see Appendix 2 for details).

Conclusions

At the initial stages of counselling it is the responsibility of the therapist to decide whether they feel they can provide a useful setting where the lesbian, gay or bisexual person can be given the support they need, and to be clear about their own attitudes, prejudices, limitations and responsibilities.

When working with single lesbian, gay and bisexual people, there are a number of factors that need to be taken into consideration. Although, on the surface, many client issues may appear similar to heterosexual problems, the therapist may well find that such preconceptions are mistaken and unless these are challenged, then the therapist will work from a disadvantage which will hinder rather than help such clients.

- There is no single, defined entity called 'The Lesbian, Gay and Bisexual Community'. Rather, there exist numerous diverse communities, based around interests, and individuals may be 'members' of one or many or none.
- Opportunities for meeting other lesbian, gay and bisexual people outside of major population centres are often extremely limited. This may result in relationships for men based solely on sexual contact and, for women, within a small, closed circle of friends and lovers. It will probably inhibit disclosure of sexual identity.
- Same sex relationship and dating skills haven't been acquired through heterosexual socialization so the development of intimacy may be difficult, especially for men. Women may find gender based expectations of their relationship styles equally unhelpful.
- Pressures to emulate certain body images can be hurtful to those outside a fashionable body stereotype. This may additionally lower self-esteem and disadvantage older people, those from ethnic and racial minorities and those with disabilities. Lesbians and gay men have different body image issues from one another and from their heterosexual counterparts as well as sharing some with them.
- Therapists can help by exploring relationship skills, recommending certain self-help books and support groups to facilitate acquisition of appropriate same sex social and relationship skills. They will need to be well informed.
- Therapists will need to interrogate their own attitudes and assumptions and their effects when meeting the diverse groups identified in this chapter, and have a duty to inform themselves as to the cultural and experiential contexts in which their clients are living.

6 | GAIL SIMON

Working with people in relationships

This chapter raises questions about the effect on therapists and clients of the dominant ideas in society about lesbian, gay and bisexual relationships. Using clinical examples from some lesbian or gay practitioners and theoretical ideas specifically from systemic and social constructionist therapy, I will discuss how therapists might expand the range and type of ideas on which they and their clients might draw. In doing so, they might move away from reproducing 'problem saturated' descriptions of gay relationships to alternatives co-created by therapist and client which liberate the individual or couple from an account of personal and collective inadequacy.

The uses of generalisations and diversity when working with lesbian, gay and bisexual couples

A few years ago, I saw an American television programme which attempted to demonstrate the effect of gender in arguing couples. The programme showed three couples arguing and concluded that of the three, the gay male couple came bottom of the table with lowest ability to communicate about their difficulties, the heterosexual couple came second because the woman made attempts to talk about their problems and the lesbian couple scored highest as they both talked openly about their disagreements.

For a while, I was reassured by this finding because it fitted with my idea of traditional women's skills but then I started to notice that my clinical work was not supporting the hypothesis that *all* lesbians in couples communicated well and *all* gay men did not. Were the couples or partners who betrayed this gender specific behaviour then the problem? Or were the findings rather limited generalisations? Perhaps generalisations can be useful as a set of ideas to draw on, but they can also be dangerous in as much as we can notice only what we are looking for and so close down opportunities for other ideas to emerge. We can, quite unwittingly, promote a description of a situation which does not fit with a couple's experience.

Therapists and their clients may resort to these generalisations in the absence of other accounts. I find it helpful to think more in terms of ideas and stories which can be a resource to all involved in therapy. White (1991: 28) says that

> It is through the narratives or the stories that persons have about their own lives and the lives of others that they make sense of their experience... these stories also largely determine which aspects of experience persons select out for expression.

As therapists and as clients we need to examine which stories we are drawing on and how they influence our thinking and actions. We also need to explore how these stories have come about and become familiar with the limits of them when working with lesbian, gay and bisexual couples.

One of the problems with writing a chapter on working with lesbian, gay or bisexual couples is the invitation to make generalisations. By making universal statements such as 'gay couples are more likely to...', one creates an idea that one can give 'true' or absolute descriptions of an apparently homogenous group of people. But the last thing a lesbian, gay or bisexual couple would want or find useful, is to be slotted into a fixed description of a 'typical' couple with an inflexible explanation of their concerns.

Generalisations do not take account of contexts. For example, we have to take other differential experience such as age, gender, culture and also ability and disadvantage into account. It is a popular misconception that because lesbians, gay men and bisexuals are different to heterosexuals we must then be similar to each other. The lesbian, gay and bisexual community is, like the heterosexual community, many communities. There are cultures within the culture. A central task in therapy, therefore, is not only valuing diversity but recognising that diversity exists (see also Chapters 2 and 5).

Relationship choices

Living with the consequences of invisibility and visibility

More in the past than the present, a number of lesbian, gay and bisexual couples emulated the gender specific behaviour of heterosexual couples with one person playing the 'man' and the other the 'woman'. There have also been couples who have not 'role played' in this way. These days many lesbians, gay men and bisexuals are not only generating more ideas about what it might mean to be a couple but also what it means to be a man or a woman or to be in a relationship.

The lesbian and gay communities have a limited range of role models to draw on because there have been fewer visible same sex relationships from earlier generations to refer to. While the odd individual may have been visible, couples rarely have been. They lived mostly in secret, as 'friends' to the outside world, sometimes even denying the nature of their involvement to each other, possibly covering up their true feelings by marrying others. For example, both Rudolph Valentino and Rock Hudson, now known to have been gay, were forced into marriage by their film studios after rumours circulated. Neither one ever 'came out' as gay and this has had implications for what biographers can tell us about their relationships. Alice B. Toklas and Gertrude Stein never explicitly acknowledged the nature of their relationship despite others knowing of their longstanding sexual partnership. These kinds of selective story-telling give distorted and excluding histories.

Perhaps the lack of visible role models from older couples is a disadvantage. The images we do have, while emblazoned with courage and humanity, often arise in the context of the dominant values of another era – of secrecy, shame and role playing, with isolation, fear and oppression taking its toll by limiting the kinds of choices which people felt able to make about their relationship lifestyles.

Heterosexual therapists who work or live in more liberal circles might be forgiven for thinking that most lesbian, gay or bisexual couples are 'out' these days and do not experience oppressive reactions. However, it is easy to forget or not realise that there are still significant numbers of people in same sex relationships who are not 'out' in some or all significant areas of their lives, i.e. with employers, colleagues, family or friends. Even today in Britain, we must remember that young men under 18 are not allowed to have sexual relationships with other men! If they do, they commit illegal 'homosexual acts'. The Church of England might tolerate 'homosexuals' but not a 'homosexual relationship' as this might involve genital contact! There are many legal, emotional, familial, economic and security reasons why couples may feel the need to keep their relationship hidden.

Being 'out' can draw discrimination too. There can be extra pressures for couples where one or both partners are 'out'. Martina Navratilova and the comedian Sandy Toksvig, for example, have recently had their relationships and families hounded by the press following their coming out. Nevertheless, they do provide images of lesbians in relationships which feel closer to the lived experience of many other couples nowadays.

There are many more families and friends these days who are prepared to work on their own feelings about sexuality and develop a genuinely warm and close relationship with someone's gay partner. Having said that, there may be some who have seemingly accepted someone's sexual orientation, but have a strong 'second wave' of anger, disgust or shame when their gay relative, colleague or friend actually starts having a sexual relationship.

There are a few couples who are not even 'out' to themselves. By this I mean that they are not describing themselves as having a lesbian, gay or bisexual relationship nor mixing with couples who do use those descriptions. There are arguments for and against labelling, of course, and perhaps it is important to consider how labels are used and by whom. For some couples, or in some contexts, naming an aspect of one's identity or status as a couple can be liberating; for others, labelling is experienced as oppressive or disqualifying in all aspects of their lives. Others find contemporary labels distasteful (see Chapters 9 and 10). What creates concern for some couples is living with the anxiety of being 'found out' by neighbours, colleagues or family or the fear that their partner will be disgusted at the use of a term and flee. This is commonly referred to as 'internalised homophobia' and will continue to make for low esteem, fear and unhappiness unless recognised and worked with. (This issue is dealt with in Chapter 3.) Simons (1991: 211) used a creative intervention with one lesbian couple where the partners were in disagreement about the nature of the relationship. She asked the more reticent partner to express her beliefs aloud in the session by saying to her partner, 'Thank God it's *you* who's the lesbian in this relationship!'

Some current issues

There may be advantages to having to create our own role models, narratives or possibilities, rather than be recruited into the idea that the only, or optimum, model of a relationship is one like that prescribed for heterosexual partnerships. Of course many heterosexual couples are now experimenting with what it means to be a woman or a man in a (heterosexual) relationship. By questioning assumptions about gender, relationships, families and marriage, lesbians, gay men and bisexuals can ask themselves what forms of relationship they want to achieve. What values are they going to place upon which relationship behaviours? How are they going to understand the role of the couple as a unit in this society or in their own cultures? Cohen (1991: 88) quotes Foucault as pointing out in 1981 that: 'The problem is not trying to find out the truth of one's sexuality within oneself, but rather, nowadays, trying to use our sexuality to achieve a variety of different types of relationships.' Doug Carl (1990: 52) in his book on same sex couples comments, 'the lack of rigid role delineation often leaves room for creativity.'

Lesbian, gay and bisexual couples are diverse in their practices and relationship structures. Some couples prefer an exclusive sexual relationship with a primary partner in the context of a long term relationship. Others may, either from the beginning of their relationship or some time into it, agree to have sexual relationships with others while remaining as primary partners. Again, each couple will decide for themselves just what this means for them. Other people will have relationships with one or a number of people which may or may not be considered to involve some form of commitment. It used to be thought that gay men were more likely to want 'open' (or polygamous) relationships and lesbians choose monogamy. However, this seems to be changing as both genders experiment with new ways of being in relationship. Perceptions of what appears to be happening currently are affected by one's own position and cultural experience – in my case as a lesbian and as a therapist with a white Jewish European experience.

Ideas about relationship practices are constantly emerging and evolving. Understandably, lesbian, gay or bisexual couples do, to a certain extent, draw on their experience of heterosexual relationships and this can be useful in determining which behaviours and arrangements they would find helpful to keep, try out or discard. But the picture we have of relationships privileges heterosexuality and certain kinds of gender roles. Carl (1990) points out that most people, including lesbians, gay men and bisexuals, carry round two ideas: first, that coupling is necessary for happiness; and second, that long term relationships are best. It is important, therefore, for same sex couples to create their own practices. To accept a given set of norms from within a society which promotes a model of personal relationships based on gender and racial inequalities and asserts certain cultural values to the exclusion of others, may mean buying too wholeheartedly into descriptions of, and beliefs about, 'normal' relationship behaviours.

Bisexual couples are extremely varied in their practices and make-up, and are subject to a number of myths. A bisexual couple might be a man and a woman, two women together or two men together. There are many couples where only one partner describes themselves as bisexual and the other as lesbian or gay or heterosexual. Many people are open with their primary partner about their bisexuality, others do not tell their partner. Some people describe themselves as bisexual and choose to be monogamous, others decide to have more than one partner of either gender. Bisexuality does not imply the need for more than one partner or for partners of both sexes simultaneously. However, a number of bisexual couples have an arrangement which allows for partners to have casual or serious relationships with others. Bisexuality is not in itself a problem. Problems are only likely to arise when couples have difficulties negotiating ground rules for their relationship, or when they encounter the prejudices of others.

There are usually questions for couples in or considering 'open' relationships which sooner or later need clarifying, about negotiating a shared vision of their relationship, how much to disclose to others (including each other) about their sexual practices or partners and agreements about safer sex practices.

Clearing the way for collaborative work with couples

It is quite possible that most heterosexual therapists will only know one or two lesbian, gay or bisexual couples socially and many might only come across lesbians, gay men and bisexuals through their work as therapists. It strikes me, therefore, that an occupational hazard of writing anything about these groups in the context of a book on therapy is that, by describing some problems lesbians, gay men and bisexuals might experience in their relationships, I might be contributing to an already problem-saturated narrative.

It is important for therapists to have a willingness to maintain a degree of uncertainty and curiosity in working with clients (Amundson *et al.* 1993). This openness creates an opportunity for the bringing forth of other 'knowledges' which couples may have or may develop with the therapist in the therapy. This is especially significant when working with couples whose relationships may be affected by stories about class, race, ability, gender, age, sexuality and so on.

Many heterosexual therapists are informed by a liberal humanist perspective of 'It is okay for you to be who *you* are'. This can translate into 'It is okay for you to be having a relationship with someone of the same sex'. What this belief tends to do is focus on the individual lesbian, gay or bisexual couple, see them as no different from heterosexual couples and encourage them to feel accepted by the therapist concerned. This acceptance is then conditional upon behaving like heterosexual couples (Kitzinger 1989). The experience of feeling obliged to 'fit in' with heterosexual culture by not rocking the dominant cultural boat ('passing') is familiar to lesbians, gay men and bisexuals (see Part I). A gay couple's description of their behaviours which might not fit with the therapist's ideals may provoke discomfort, impatience and disapproval in the therapist and a retreat to more stereotypical beliefs about lesbian, gay and bisexual 'psychology'. Couples who do not fit with the therapist's ideas may then be constructed as difficult or disturbed, deviating from the therapist's idea of a 'normal' lesbian, gay and bisexual couple! (Kitzinger 1989).

Treating the couple as an individualised unit without locating their experience in the lesbian, gay and bisexual communities is likely to contribute to a sense of isolation, deviance and disturbance, so reinforcing the negative stories prevalent in society about same sex relationships. Disagreements in the couple about what it means to be having a relationship or how to conduct one are often seen solely in the context of those two people and their life histories. Their experiences could additionally be thought of in the wider systems of other social contexts and groupings so that they are relocated in both the personal and the political arena (Kitzinger 1989; Simon forthcoming). This is a difficulty for most therapists, however they define their sexual orientation, so I will make some suggestions about how to work with the notion of wider systems later on.

Obviously the descriptions we come up with as therapists will depend on the range of ideas that we have at our disposal. More importantly, we have to work with the couple to explore the meanings they are giving to the occurrence of a problem. Having said this, there are many occasions when I hear lesbians or gay men describe their problems in terms that sound as if they have been absorbed from a textbook: two women: 'We seem to be merged'; two men: 'We are having difficulty dealing with our feelings'.

It is not uncommon for lesbian, gay and bisexual couples to be talking in the very language which seeks to disqualify their experience. In order to help couples move away from inherited descriptions, one might need to work with them to deconstruct their thinking. These are some questions that I have found useful with couples to trace the development of their narrative and open up the possibility of re-description by the couple, which is likely to contextualise their behaviours and so take them outside of a pathologising discourse.

- What has happened in the couple that they notice they have 'difficulty dealing with their feelings'?
- Who else thinks this?
- Who would disagree with this idea?
- Are there times and circumstances when they do not have 'difficulty dealing with their feelings'?
- What are the differences in the circumstances that give rise to different descriptions of their behaviour?
- How have they come to be recruited into this description of their experience?
- If they were each to find another way of describing this problem, what would they say?

Why do lesbian, gay and bisexual couples come for therapy?

Having practised as a therapist for over 10 years with heterosexual, lesbian, gay and bisexual individuals, couples and families, I am drawing on my experience with over 150 same sex or bisexual couples with whom I have worked. Two-thirds have been lesbians, just under a third were gay males, there were about 10 families and four male/female bisexual couples. Fifteen per cent of couples I have seen have been of mixed race. I have also worked with many more lesbians and gay men individually who are, or have been, in relationships. This work has occurred primarily in a private lesbian and gay counselling practice where clients would know that I am a lesbian. I have also worked in other counselling settings with all sections of the population where clients would not necessarily be aware of my 'sexual identity'.

Couples present with a range of issues. Common descriptions include:

- concern over an increase in rows;
- couple feels communication has broken down and they are drifting apart;
- one partner wants 'more space', the other is worried;
- conflict over status of relationship;
- at least one partner is or has been involved with someone else;
- decisions about living together;
- decisions about having children and parenting issues;
- separating partners working at a positive end or transition;
- decline or changes in sexual relationship;
- violence between partners.

Additional issues affecting couples presenting for counselling:

- effect of work pressures on relationship;
- inflexible communication patterns;
- change in meaning of common interests or relationship;
- cross-cultural issues regarding values, understandings or power imbalance based on race, or other factors;
- renegotiation or clarification of what partners want from relationship;
- jealousy, insecurity and/or isolation;
- relationship with families;
- coming out issues;
- living with HIV status or other health concerns.

What do you think about these lists? Do you perceive there to be similarities and differences between what heterosexual and lesbian, gay or bisexual couples might experience as problematic? Are some of these issues more likely to be experienced in some sections of the population than others?

Bearing in mind the emergence of, and participation in, a critical discourse about relationship practices, lesbian, gay and bisexual couples rarely recognise the *pioneering* element in their relationships. Problems they have are often interpreted according to the old adage that gay relationships are unsuccessful, rather than seen as problems anyone might expect to come across at certain points in a relationship and especially where proceeding without clear guidelines.

Case examples in this chapter are not taken exclusively from any one particular couple. I have used examples of situations which I have come across in a similar form on several occasions. Where conversation is a direct quotation from a session, permission from the clients has been sought.

Case example 1
Anna and Bianca had been together for four years and lived together for three and a half years. They came to counselling as they were rowing and uncertain about the future of their relationship.

They started living together after five months when Bianca moved in with Anna as she had to leave her accommodation. Bianca was now wanting to move out, complaining they were 'merged' and saying she needed more space. Anna was fearful that Bianca was ending the relationship.

Anna: I am scared that if we don't live together, we won't be a couple.
Bianca: But that's like the heterosexual idea that if we don't live together, it means we're breaking up.
Anna: People have already said that we have broken up because we are living apart. It makes me wonder if we have...
Bianca: But we haven't! We just haven't got a label for it.

This is a couple struggling to create their own norms without being intimidated by the many voices around them. By taking the idea of 'couple' out of the heterosexual framework (Hall 1987) and trying to bring their own meaning to their relationship, they are expanding the choices they can make rather than fearing 'inevitable' consequences of certain actions. They are exploring and inventing their own ways of 'relationshipping' and not necessarily operating within a particular kind of idea of 'relationship progression'; this might culminate in living apart as opposed to living together.

The description of 'merged' which Bianca gives is best thought of as an umbrella term, borrowed from American feminist psychology (Burch 1982; Mencher 1990) which explores alternative ways of thinking about patterns of attachment between women, more specifically in the context of lesbian relationships. Despite attempts by these theorists to reframe separation and attachment issues positively, many lesbians use this description to criticise their relationship. I have found that there is almost never any form of identity confusion or inability to be apart when people use this term. Togetherness does not seem to be a problem but negotiating change in how they spend their time often is. This is especially the case where couples have a limited frame of reference for 'healthy relationships' and bring too many negative interpretations to change-over-time in their relationship. Concern about 'merged-ness' usually comes at a time in a relationship where certain patterns have come to dominate and the couple are nervous about renegotiating.

Another most unhelpful myth amongst lesbians (and some other couples) is that they move in together too quickly and that this is something to be embarrassed about. Where couples do choose to live together soon after becoming involved with each other, it often seems to coincide with a need for one partner to change accommodation. I have particularly noticed this where partners are renting or on low incomes so I am inclined, in many cases, to connect these decisions with housing availability or economics rather than with sexual orientation or relationship patterns.

Case example 2
David, 36, a businessman, and Eddie, 32, a musician, had been involved for about eight years, living together for nearly seven. The first year of their relationship was spent commuting between different towns at weekends. Then Eddie came up to London to take a full time degree course. He met David's friends and became part of that social circle. Eddie found an uncomfortable bedsit for a few months and then moved in with David when David bought a house. Around this time, David got a promotion which involved often being away on business. Eddie found sessional work as a musician. Both had been diagnosed as HIV positive prior to getting involved with each other. They came to counselling as they had been rowing and had not been getting on.

David: I work really hard during the week so we can have a home and then I get home, I'm exhausted and the place is deserted and it's a mess. I can't relax if the place is untidy and washing needs hanging up.
Eddie: I can't take being criticised by you all the time.
David: But it's not like you don't have any time.
Eddie: You know I have to practice. But it's true, I could do more. I just got carried away on Friday and went for a drink with John afterwards.
David: But it isn't just this Friday, it's every week and it's especially bad when I've been away for a few days. I think he is out the whole time I'm away.
Eddie: So?
David: He doesn't eat properly or get enough sleep. We agreed to live healthily and keep our T-cell counts up but he just wants to rave around the clock...
Eddie: I want to live a life.
David: I ring and he's not there. I end up sitting in a hotel bedroom in a foreign town and wonder where he is.
Therapist: You worry because...?
David: Because he's not looking after himself.
Eddie: He thinks I'm meeting other guys.
David: Are you? [pause]

Eddie: [to therapist] This is what happens. We row. I admit I am in the wrong. We go out to eat and it's OK again.
David: For a while.

There could have been several things going on here. Let's speculate:

1 This couple had always had time apart imposed on them by where they lived or by David's work trips. Perhaps they had never negotiated ground rules. Or perhaps they had maintained the same expectations about seeing each other when they could, which Eddie was now challenging.
2 For years Eddie had waited for David to come home and had been the penniless student for a long time; now he had a job, more status and different priorities.
3 David has been very health conscious. The pressure of his work made him particularly concerned about taking good care of himself. Being concerned about each other's health and T-cell counts had been an important and loving part of their relationship. Eddie's work brought out another side of him. He felt excited by his new found recognition outside of the relationship and associated care about his health with domestic routine.
4 Eddie was keen to socialise and have more of his own friends. David was happy to carry on seeing his friends as a couple and to come home after work and flop.
5 Maybe something else had happened recently, like a bereavement, which prompted each man to review his priorities.

In circumstances similar to David and Eddie's, where couples have not clarified expectations from early on, I have found some ideas from the Coordinated Management of Meaning (Pearce 1989) valuable in exploring the relationship between patterns of thinking and behaviour. This 'strange loop' (Pearce 1989) shows how a couple might go round in circles with potential beliefs helping to maintain the pattern of relating.

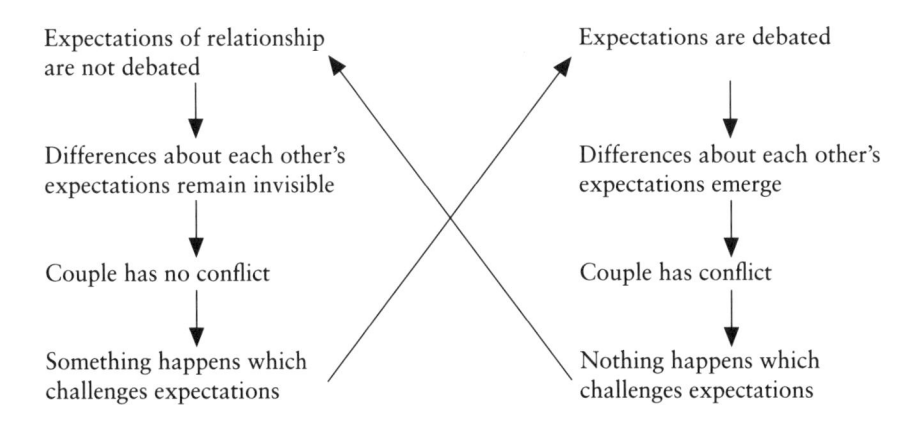

Expectations of relationship are not debated
↓
Differences about each other's expectations remain invisible
↓
Couple has no conflict
↓
Something happens which challenges expectations

Expectations are debated
↓
Differences about each other's expectations emerge
↓
Couple has conflict
↓
Nothing happens which challenges expectations

There will be beliefs which hold such loops in place. By uncovering them and connecting them to the loop, there is the possibility of deconstructing them with clients, so opening up further options.

Beliefs maintaining this 'strange loop' might be:

- 'Talking makes things worse' (an idea from family or life experience);
- 'Gay people should just be able to have good relationships without having to spell everything out' (a myth from heterosexual culture where there appear to be clear rules for successful relationships which some believe do not need clarifying);
- 'Identifying differences makes for conflict. Conflict ends in violence' (a family or life experience story);
- 'Gay relationships are doomed anyway' (an idea from heterosexual culture leaving the couple feeling there is no point in them trying to resolve difficulties).

Case example 3
Liz and Fran had an initial consultation to discuss differences in their sexual desires which they were very worried about. In the consultation, we explored their patterns of communicating and their thinking about 'normal' sexual behaviour. I positively connoted their differences as diversity to be valued and encouraged them to share their ideas about their own sexuality with each other.

A month later, the couple returned for the follow up consultation. Fran said she felt reassured after the last session. It turned out that she had been worried about them 'getting things right'. She had been amazed at the insight that it was OK for them to do things 'their way' and whatever suited them as a couple. Liz agreed, saying she had been a bit worried about what other people would think of them as a lesbian couple as lesbians have to be more perfect. To admit to difficulties said something negative about lesbians.

The clients are starting to deconstruct the powerful disqualifying story of 'lesbian failure' which has been acting as a frame for interpreting their experiences and influencing their thoughts about what lesbians can and cannot do, i.e. 'lesbian couples cannot have problems because it would confirm a negative stereotype of lesbian relationships'.

They are also deconstructing received ideas about 'sex' which Hall (1990) saw as an umbrella term for many varied practices; she asked lesbians thoroughly to review their own ideas about what 'sex' is. This is a controversial point in lesbian communities as some would argue that lesbian sexuality has always been denied or underplayed. Others argue that 'sex' as we have come to know it, is a male construct which refers to a heterosexual male experience in a gender-laden context and bears little relation to lesbian experience which needs major re-description, probably involving new terms and the creation of a fresh epistemology.

In circles of younger women and men, who may have less access to older sections of the community, couples who have been together any length of time are held up as role models which can bring extra pressure to those couples. A similar dynamic is described in respect of lesbian and gay parenting in Chapter 7.

Case example 4
Connie and Jeanine, age 23 and 24, had been together for two and a half years when they came to counselling. They felt stuck and on the verge of splitting up. They felt resentful of the one-way support to their friends in the small town where they lived.

> *Connie*: The longer we stay together, the more everyone else idealises us and the less we talk to friends about our problems. Or even to each other.
> *Jeanine*: We bought into the idea ourselves. [shaking her head] 'What, *us* go to couple counselling?'!
> *Therapist*: So how would your friends describe you as a couple?
> *Connie*: They just see our strengths. I feel a failure.
> *Jeanine*: People are asking why we aren't together so much now.

They have bought into an idea of longer = better and better = conflict-free. It turns out that they had rarely rowed. Connie had wanted to argue but felt angry behaviour was not something that feminists should resort to. This prohibition fitted neatly with Jeanine's dislike of rows from experiences in her family. In addition, they feared letting down the lesbian community and destroying the picture of them as an 'ideal couple' by acknowledging they had problems and needed help. Despite being 'out' and having many lesbian friends, I see this couple as being isolated in another type of closet where they were experiencing censorship and restriction in their choices about how they might wish to be a couple and in choosing which images of their relationship to portray. (Living in a small town adds another important dimension, as discussed in Chapter 5.)

I asked them some *wider system* questions (Simon forthcoming), to help them find validity for their experiences in a group beyond their immediate friends, families and counsellor.

- 'If we could, by magic, skip to the next town in this county, what do you think the chances are of finding another couple in a similar position to yourselves?'
- 'Supposing we hold a conference now for all the lesbian and gay couples in a similar position to you from smaller towns across the UK, what kinds of things would these couples be putting on the agenda?'

- 'What effect would it have on you two, as a couple, to be surrounded by so many other lesbian or gay couples in a similar position?'
- 'Imagine you have two or three days at this conference and you are now returning to your home town, to your friends, what do you think you might do differently?'

By using a *hypothetical audience* (Simon forthcoming) (the 'conference' of other couples) with *wider system/context questions* we are drawing on a range of experience which might not otherwise find a voice or an audience and hence, validation. Another advantage to using these questions is that the counsellor does not need to be an expert in the area of the client's concerns. The couple find their own solutions and at the same time relocate their experience into a more public or political arena.

Final reflections

Having said that lesbian, gay or bisexual couples must create their own models of relationships and make their own choices both within and outside of the dominant culture, we are trying to do this while constantly facing negativity, ignorance and threats across many areas of our lives. This occurs, for example, in the area of people's career and employment opportunities or the right to custody of one's own children or even just walking down the street together. Consequently, many couples who are happily 'out' amongst gay and gay affirmative friends, may work hard to appear a very 'normal', conforming couple (i.e. with heterosexual values and roles) in the public settings of the courts or the work place so as to meet the expectations of others with the power to hire and fire or determine custody orders.

It is not easy for lesbian, gay and bisexual couples immediately to provide an alternative framework or language. They have also been brought up in the modernist tradition of non-participant expertise. By this I mean that heterosexual professionals have developed theories about lesbians, gay men and bisexuals with whom they have little experience except, periodically, as patients. Meaning has been imposed on to gay people's experiences, desires and behaviours and these meanings have become theories or 'truths' which often support the philosophy of elitist institutions (see Chapter 1). To quote Kathleen Stacey (1993: 11):

> Adherence to a post-modern sensibility provides constant challenges to one's construction of the world as a therapist, with an expectation to operate within multiple realities, to develop a heightened and refined social consciousness and the ability to detect and elucidate the discourses which dominate the production of meaning in our world.

The dominant cultures within which we are all living are not inclined to encourage the emergence of new and alternative ideas and descriptions of lesbian, gay and bisexual experiences. It is vitally important that other 'voices' are heard, find validation and participate in the forming of different ways of thinking about ourselves and our relationships, so increasing the choices available to couples and validating their experiences.

Conclusions

- Therapeutic work will benefit if therapists can be curious about dominant ideas and generalisations about couples and about gay relationships, whether these ideas come from clients or research, or from therapeutic literature or the therapist.
- Therapeutic openness allows new 'knowledge' to emerge.
- There are few visible models of successful lesbian, gay or bisexual relationships and 'success' can be understood in different ways.
- Therapists and clients can together re-describe relationships and beliefs about them which liberate all involved from accounts of inadequacy or pathology.
- Comparisons between normative models of heterosexual relationships and lesbian, gay and bisexual ones are unhelpful, often heterosexist and do not take account of the pioneering element involved in the latter.
- Pressures to subscribe to prescriptive, or demanding narratives within their own communities may lead gay couples to fear disclosures of difficulties and fail to find support for working issues through.
- Issues surrounding safety and opportunity will make being 'out' or not highly significant within relationships.
- In trying not to discomfort therapists, clients may try to pass for dominant culture couples as near as possible who do not locate difficulties within wider contexts of relationship development generally, and their social and political settings.
- Examples of *wider system* approaches have been given.

7 | HELENA HARGADEN AND SARA LLEWELLIN

Lesbian and gay parenting issues

Parenting is a core human issue which will be raised in some guise within the therapeutic relationship whoever the client. For lesbians and gay men the issues involved in whether or how to become parents, how to raise children, and how to choose and/or grieve for not having children, will be significantly different from those raised in a heterosexual context. Issues facing bisexual clients will be different again.

This chapter outlines some of the homophobic prejudices which lesbian and gay clients confront in approaching parenting, gives examples of lesbian and gay involvement with parenting and raises specific issues arising from such circumstances for clients. It provides therapists with information on supporting non-traditional families. Because bisexuals are likely to have issues about parenting only in respect of the 'same sex' dimension of their sexuality, the emphasis here is on lesbian and gay sexualities.

The very important place of gay and bisexual men in relation to child care is as neglected an area of focus as it is in a heterosexual context; the denial of men's significant roles as parents and child carers is widespread in western culture and worsened when attached to common prejudices about homosexual males or those supporting a single model of what a 'family' might be.

Prerequisites for working well with gay, lesbian and bisexual clients are to have brought into awareness our own potentially harmful prejudicial attitudes and beliefs and to be well informed. In respect of parenting issues, we need to look at the common prejudices held in western culture about gay men and lesbians in relation to children and check out their influences upon ourselves. We also need some general information about options and difficulties facing bisexuals, lesbians and gay men who have, or who want, children.

Any of a wide range of concerns may present in our consulting room. We cannot have, and do not need, in-depth information to cover every eventuality. We simply need an idea of the options and obstacles and how lesbian and gay experiences are different in the world than those of heterosexual people.

Background

Some parenting matters have a universal human quality: how, when, whether, and with whom to have children; how best to care for those children; how to manage the extraordinary demands of parenthood; how to cope with infertility; how to integrate children into adult lives.

All of these issues have subtly different meanings in any culture according to its governing principles and norms. A culture based on principles of collectivism will approach these questions very differently to one based on individualism. A culture with belief in an afterlife will have significantly different attitudes to parenting than one espousing an existentialist view; one with a fearsome deity than one with a benign deity; one steeped in poverty than one of plenty; one with minority status than one with majority.

Values and assumptions which lie behind the way people approach questions of parenting have contextual as well as cultural specificity. For example, in times of war or other crisis, norms or general practices may be adapted or abandoned in the interests of expediency. In Britain during World War II, for example, women were required for the work force; therefore nursery provision was the norm and sexual mores underwent a radical change. Likewise, legislation in areas of social policy will create or deny individual choices. Housing, matrimonial, civil rights, welfare and other laws will all affect people's life choices.

Key social and political changes have come about as a result of sociopolitical movements since the mid-1960s. Procreation, the right to control fertility, and a critique of the nuclear family have all been important to feminist, black and gay liberation movements.

When white feminists began to say in large numbers 'we have the right to control (i.e. limit) our fertility by means of contraception, abortion, choice', black, 'third world' and disabled women responded with 'we have the right *not* to have our fertility controlled (i.e. limited) by forced contraception and sterilization, prejudicial medical care, lack of access to housing and money'.

These related perspectives have influenced conscious choices for lesbians, black and white, in respect of fertility. For some, the choice *not* to have children is an important element of lesbian identity. Some go further and suggest that motherhood is an enslaving and limited construct, the cornerstone of women's oppression. Certainly therapists need critically to unravel the relationship between caretaking, caring, nurturing and gender, if they are to be effective with parents or prospective parents. Many other lesbians, especially since the late 70s and early 80s, have approached the question of motherhood from the position of entitlement *to* parenthood rather than freedom from it, and increasingly gay men are asserting their own right to parent.

Why parent?

This is a valid and useful question to ask of anyone about to embark upon parenthood. For many, becoming a parent is a major life aspiration or expectation, and being a parent a major life responsibility. It will be intimately bound up with our social and gender identity, self-perception and public persona, as well as with our own history and experience as children. For lesbians or gay men, it may be something previously denied as an option which now seems possible. Even so, your client may want to explore why and whether parenthood is attractive to them, why now and the practical and psychological aspects of how to go ahead.

The affirmative therapist is not looking for justifications, but rather for a genuine exploration of the issues: creativity, readiness, desire, identity, practical capacity. They will be aware that the experience of lesbians and gay men wanting children is that of being constantly questioned and expected to have more well-defined answers than heterosexuals. Our situations demand (and usefully) that gay people ask themselves these questions. However, the therapist's questioning may be experienced as oppressive if it mirrors the responses of family, mainstream culture and friends. Your client may find it useful if you make some reference to understanding the basic issues they face with regard to entitlement. A simple humorous reference to the fact that heterosexual couples might never consider the question could reassure clients that you assume their equal right.

'The map'

There are no cultural norms or social structures for parenting other than heterosexual ones. Lesbians and gay men having children have to make it up as they go along. There is a body of experience to be tapped from women and (much smaller) men who have already done it, and this is useful to a degree (see Appendix 2). Lesbian and gay parents lose track of the numbers of others who have sought us out to ask us about our own families and how we came by them. The lack of formula is both a pressure and liberation, requiring proactive problem solving and encouraging autonomy (see Gail Simon's discussion of new possibilities for same sex relationships in Chapter 6).

At the psychological level, however, the lack of a 'map', or points of reference, may leave the client's 'inner child' feeling lonely, frightened or confused. The skilled therapist will understand this and provide the holding and protection needed for the client.

It will be valuable to explore feelings (and practical issues) about lifestyle choices and the shape of the family. If this is a single parent venture have the practical and psychological implications of that been explored? If it is a couple venture are both partners equally keen or is there some disparity and tension? Same sex couples will need to pay attention to their expectations of each other in respect of roles and responsibilities in ways which heterosexual couples are much less likely to. The therapist should not assume that the model offered by the heterosexual family will suffice (as indeed it no longer does for many heterosexuals). Lesbian couples must decide who will bear the child, or who first? What level of commitment is the other partner making to the child and to the mother? If it is a full parental commitment, what pre-agreements can be made to cover the possible eventuality of relationship breakdown? Male couples also need to work through and agree areas of responsibility and commitment, roles in child care and employment, and best arrangements in the eventuality of separation or death. Far better to have some principles established when the relationship is functioning than to have to attend to them when in crisis. Maintenance, inheritance of joint property or debt (including possibly the home), access and parental control... how will these be handled in unconventional relationships which do not have the sanction of state and law?

Common prejudices

What do they have to do with us?

First, we need to be aware of, and name embedded prejudices about gay people and children in order to make sense of beliefs about lesbians and gay men as parents. Deep-seated fear and disgust underpin these projective fantasies and these are then rationalized. Second, therapists need to critically examine their own responses to images of lesbians and gay men with children or as parents and understand them in the context of cultural as well as personal beliefs. Third, naming and understanding these prejudices informs us about the lives and psychological experiences of lesbians and gay men, enabling us to be more empathic and challenging as clinicians. Fourth, uncovering fears and fantasies beneath the rationalizations will be necessary in addressing the negative beliefs the client may have been recruited into and have internalized.

The most commonly held prejudice is that gay people should not be allowed to work or to live with children because they are child molesters (especially gay men with boys) or they would be a bad influence on children (i.e. might make them gay). There is, of course, no evidence to support these prejudices, which few therapists would identify as personal beliefs. Nevertheless, they are frequently part of the cultural belief system by which we have been influenced. We will carry vestiges of belief in them, even when our current adult thinking contradicts them.

Importantly, misogynistic and homophobic arguments against lesbians or gay men having relationships with children, whilst originating from mainstream culture are also experienced at an individual level. Lesbian or gay clients will not be wholly free from self-contempt, self-denial or self-repression. For this reason more than any other, it is vital that, as therapist, you have brought your negative opinions and feelings into consciousness, whatever your own sexuality. Repressed or denied prejudices will always 'out' at some level, and be relayed to the client with axiomatically damaging consequences. In working through the following common objections to gay people parenting, it will be important to address gender assumptions along with those attaching to sexuality.

It is not natural

This argument may be motivated by religion or biological determinism, or sexism, all of which have been used through history to restrict (usually women's) control over fertility. For many people 'natural' is synonymous with heterosexual. In particular, western culture is obsessed with 'the sex act' and its romantic product – the child. Therefore the mechanics of conception have a focal significance in social control and romantic thinking as well as psychological theory, and it is this that is named 'natural'. Chapters 1 and 3 include discussion on the origins of such ideas in relation to sexuality and their damaging impact on us all. Of course the reality is that many ways in which we control our environment are not natural and most of us would be hard put to define what we meant by the term or how we would relate it to human progress. Conceiving naturally is seen as sacrosanct while immunizing unnaturally against disease, for example, is prized by most people.

A child needs a male and a female parent

Linked to notions of natural and normal and heavily reinforced by psychoanalytic theories, this argument is a defence of the known and the romantic. It supposes the western nuclear family to be ideal and the norm, when arguably it is neither. It is not the family in which most children grow up, and neither is it the only structure in which they flourish. In many cultures women are the primary caretakers of children and the male nurturing role is severely limited. Those subscribing to ideas that males and females have markedly different functions as caregivers will be concerned by proposals for children to have two parents of one gender. The influences of Freudianism must not be underestimated and some familiarity with a critique of the Freudian tradition would be useful to any therapist working in areas of sexuality, child development and gender.

A boy needs a male role model

This argument is often posited on the supposition that adolescent boys without fathers become anti-social teenagers or become 'like women' (effeminate, or gay). It is by no means proved that the absence of a father is the major critical component. There are many male role models for boys to choose, and many of them are poor ones. Providing good male role models for boys (and girls!) if it is important, is important for *all*. Interestingly, the very idea of a male 'role model' runs counter to the 'nature' argument; if you have to learn how to be a man, then manliness is learnt behaviour. Nature dictates that a boy will become a man... the cultural anxiety is fear about what *sort* of man. Alan Sinfield's *The Wilde Century* (1994) includes substantial material on the history of fear of 'effeminacy' in Britain.

Gay parents will make their children gay

This concern arises from prejudices about sexuality and the affirmative response would be 'so what?' Studies to date indicate otherwise (Golombok *et al.* 1983; Green *et al.* 1986). Children growing up in lesbian households have been found in these studies to be no more likely to be homosexual than children raised in heterosexual households and clinical evidence suggests the same for children raised in gay male families. Almost all lesbians, gay and bisexual people grow up in nominally heterosexual families and in a determinedly heterosexual environment (see Chapter 1 for discussion of homosexual incidence).

It is selfish to have children just because you want to

Some heterosexual people say this without being able to hear that what they are actually saying is, 'We don't want you to have the freedoms and choices we have.' Interestingly, heterosexuals can be accused of being selfish if they *don't* want children. The logical extension of this argument is that it would be ideal if all children were conceived by accident!

It is not fair on the children

Some will argue that it is unfair on children consciously to put them in the position of being different. It used to be heard as an argument against mixed race marriages. Claims that children will be embarrassed or confused usually come from people who are themselves embarrassed or confused. An example from our experience is when some people, hearing our sons referring to us both as their mummies, saw this as evidence that they were confused. In fact, the boys are not remotely confused; they have two mummies – just as other kids might have two grandmas or two dogs. The confusion was that of the onlooker. Children clearly need to know how to protect themselves from other people's hostility, disbelief or mere surprise. While this may not be 'fair', it can be growthful rather than harmful if handled by competent parents. Nor is it only the children of gay parents who have to learn about prejudices and difference in this way. It is homophobia which is most unfair to such families and which the therapist working affirmatively will be prepared to address.

Bringing children into same sex relationships

Large numbers of lesbians and gay men have children, and it is useful to chart the routes by which this comes about. There will be a different set of psychological considerations for each individual as always in the therapeutic situation. There will also be social meanings and pressures on lesbians and gay men in each of the following situations, requiring choices and responses which are different to those of their heterosexual counterparts.

Lesbians with children from previous heterosexual unions

Some women establish lesbian identities after being actively heterosexual. This may be because they had never before had the opportunity to explore their erotic feelings towards women. It may be because they have decided heterosexual relationships are too unequal to want to carry on with. It may be that they are bisexual or simply 'fell in love' with a particular woman. There is no pattern. It is a perfectly normal occurrence on the spectrum of sexual development discussed in the first chapter of this book. As mothers, however, women in this position will face difficulties which may present in a therapeutic relationship. Particular issues might include: responding to the reactions of ex-partners and children, forming new relationships and dealing with social hostility.

Gay men with children from previous heterosexual unions

Lots of gay and bisexual men live in heterosexual families, some 'out' and some closeted. Some men do not realize their sexual identity when they marry, some develop their gayness after they marry, and some know they are gay (or bisexual) and do not want to live in a publicly unconventional way. Thus many gay men have children in heterosexual unions. The issues for the individual will depend on:

- whether they stay in the relationship or leave it;
- whether they come out to the spouse, and her response;
- whether they come out to the children, and their response;
- their own relationship to their sexuality.

Gay men are very vulnerable if the children's mother is hostile, homophobic or hurt in any combination. Their relationships with, and access to, their children can be easily compromised or obstructed. This is partly due to sexist prejudice about men and child care in general but much exacerbated by homophobic attitudes towards the involvement of gay men with children. Few men have preferred court orders to private negotiations, even where simple access is concerned. Time will tell whether the Children Act (1989) has a beneficial impact on this in the future (see above).

Among the issues which may arise in counselling are:

- the internal struggle over whether to 'come out' and the risks this involves (see Chapter 4) and the intrapsychic process connected to loss of a presumed heterosexuality;
- dealing with the virulent homophobia which surrounds gay men in relation to (especially male) children as well as cultural prejudices against men caring for children without women;
- the negotiation skills needed to maintain the right to an active relationship with the child(ren) and dealing with social services, the law, the wider family, schools, etc.;
- the parenting skills and personal resources needed to support the children through the trauma and change, especially with no role models or support systems;
- the impact of new partners (his or hers) and their interrelating with the child(ren);
- the loss of access to children where this is the outcome and the resulting anger and grief.

Ex-partners' reactions

These can be emotionally difficult in any circumstances and especially fraught where there are children involved. As in any break-up, children can become the weapons with which adult battles are fought. For lesbians, however, there is a real possibility of a custody battle in which they will be subjected to great intrusion into their personal lives. Until recently women lost custody in a significant proportion of these cases. This is now not the usual outcome, although still possible (see Appendix 3 for useful reading). There are potential benefits for lesbian mothers in the Children

Act (1989), which obviates the need for a custody judgement in every case and emphasizes cooperative arrangements, thus discouraging battles of pride.

Some ex-partners give the children powerful messages that their mother's sexuality is problematic, and thereby make it so. This is more likely to have negative impact on the child's sexual development than the sexuality of those who parent them. Occasionally ex-partners will go so far as to 'out' the woman in places she would have chosen to remain undeclared, thus creating a sense of insecurity for the children and their mother. This may then be used as evidence of the lack of stability in the home life which she is providing.

Children's reactions

Children's responses are influenced by such factors as age, psychological and emotional states, gender, value systems, loyalty to their father, the father's reaction, the quality of family life (both prior and on offer), the degree of material change to which they are exposed (e.g. loss of income, drop in standards of living, the requirement to change schools or uproot) and whether they are already familiar with non-traditional families and gay people.

Many children have objections or reservations normal in the process of change. It may be difficult for the people involved to hear the child rather than what they perceive to be homophobia, although the child's prejudices also need to be worked through. The child's need to be supported through a period of trauma can be in conflict with the mother's need to define herself. A skilled therapist will help the mother to hear and acknowledge the child rather than dismiss or deny their responses.

Children may feel disloyal to someone whatever they do. They may not have enough information to understand what is going on. They might not have any strategy for dealing with their friends or school. They can resent becoming 'unusual' when they have not been before. They may feel jealous of, or misplaced by, a new passion whether that be a person or a new identity. They may simply feel powerless at not being the people who make, or even influence, decisions. The woman will need permission to be herself, together with support and protection if she is to facilitate her children expressing their emotional response healthily.

Not all children respond negatively by any means. Most respond with complexity and some are unequivocally supportive. For most, loyalty to their mother and the sense of security this engenders stand them in good stead. As with any other crisis or change, children who are held in boundaried structures and unconditionally loved and listened to will adapt to new situations and learn to embrace them. Therapists working with families and children can play a key role in all these circumstances.

New relationships

There are stresses in the formation of any new family constellation. These circumstances are compounded by the lack of expected social structures or role models. Much will depend upon the new lover, her experience and attitudes, and how these interplay with the emergent lesbian identity and established parental identity of the mother. Your client, of course, may be either of these people or, if you work with couples, both.

There may be rivalry between partner and children for the attention of the mother. The new lover may have little experience of children or more experience than the mother or find the demands which parenthood places upon the relationship difficult. In some instances, she may seek to compromise the relationship between mother and children or make observations about their relationships which are painful to hear and difficult to handle.

The role and identity of the new partner will need to be negotiated. She was not there from the beginning and the children (usually) have another parent, their father. She may however, take on responsibilities for the rearing and supporting of the family. Who is she then, in the public and even in the private domain? Does she have a very different approach to raising children? Does she have, or has she had and lost, children herself? Does she have a longstanding lesbian identity which challenges, and is challenged by, the new relationship? How will this new couple organize time, money, sex-life, physical space, holidays, extended families?

Outside influences

The psychological impact of social hostility should not be underestimated, even where the client is not exploring it. Sources of specific tension may be: colleagues, grandparents, church, school, children's peer groups and the respective friendship circles of the new partners. Any or all of these may project their fantasies onto the new situation, especially in relation to the children. The client will need help to deal with unhelpful responses from others. How will this new family derive support from friends and the wider family, as well as from the communities in which they live and work, in order to ensure their success? The covert prejudices conveyed by others' responses will be difficult to explore unless the therapist has examined their own; the hardest prejudices to spot are those you share.

Having children within same sex relationships

Issues of generation

Lesbians and gay men wanting children have to contend with a range of feelings, including anger and grief, about the fact that they are unable in their own loving sexual relationships to generate children. Arriving at the most suitable alternative from the range of options presently available will depend upon practical issues (availability, situation), personal ones (preferences, beliefs) and emotional ones. In all instances, there is a need to guard against potential health hazards including HIV transmission. There follows a summary of the choices for lesbians and those for gay men (see Appendix 2 for further information).

The options for lesbians

Anonymous artificial insemination by donor (AID) through a clinic

The majority of private clinics provide services exclusively for married couples. Pregnancy Advisory Service (PAS) is the only one to state unequivocally that they do not discriminate against lesbian customers, and they only operate in London. Other clinics say they assess each case on merit. Whether this means equal scrutiny with heterosexuals is not clear and presumably depends on the attitudes of the interviewers or owners.

The principle of the welfare of the child is important in the Human Fertilization and Embryology Bill, which is the governing document of the licensing body for fertility clinics. While important as an ethical principle, clearly individual interpretation will be vulnerable to prejudice.

AID via a clinic is expensive, especially if conception does not take place quickly (currently around £200 consultation followed by £100 per menstrual cycle). Clinics usually have a conservative upper age limit, few taking on women over 38. The methodology involves the deep freezing of the sperm. Anecdotal evidence strongly suggests that for potency, 'fresh is best'.

On the plus side, the health and infection screening in the clinics is good, once you have been accepted the process is straightforward and, if genuine paternal anonymity is preferred, by this method it is (as yet) guaranteed.

Anonymous donor self insemination (SI)

Self insemination is the preferred choice of women who want no involvement from the father at all and cannot afford a clinic. The donor produces sperm into a clean receptacle and a go-between keeps it warm and delivers it to the receiver, who puts it into her vagina using a 10ml syringe without the needle. There need be no medical mystique; it is a simple, straightforward technique. Finding a donor can be difficult, especially for black women. It is best done by joining a network in your nearest big city, or by advertising. Often gay men are preferred as donors, or more amenable to contributing in this way to same sex parenting.

Known donor self insemination

Some lesbians prefer to know the donor. This may be a trusted friend or a known donor with whom there is no established relationship. Either way the motive is usually for the child to have the opportunity to know, and perhaps to have a relationship with, the father. All parties need to be clear what they will and will not provide and whether they are open to further negotiation. The method is as above, except both parties can be in the same building and no go-between is needed. A lesbian may choose to be inseminated by her partner as an act symbolic of their shared intention.

Heterosexual sex

Some lesbians have 'affairs' or 'one night stands' with men in order to conceive. While this has the appeal of simplicity, it is very haphazard and can be risky in terms of health, safety and self-respect. Psychological implications will need to be explored.

The options for gay men

Many men actively want children, gay men among them. Indeed in the past the desire for fatherhood has propelled lots of gay men into unsuitable marriages and denial of their own sexuality, with unhappy consequences. Although still relatively unusual, there are some ways in which gay men are becoming parents today and remaining authentic. There is also increasing debate about the issues involved. Gay male parents will encounter multiple discrimination. Western industrial societies have not supported men as child carers and the gay communities are not yet radically different in attitudes. Some gay men, like some lesbians, regard childlessness as an asset and it is fair to say that most gay male lifestyles do not accommodate childrearing. There are few venues, care facilities, child-friendly spaces or activities and few support systems available.

Common prejudices attaching to homosexuality and contact with children will be exacerbated in the case of men when it is seen as 'natural' for women to want, even to need, children and not so for men and where women are endowed with (often unwanted) assumed parental qualities or skills unavailable to men.

As with their lesbian counterparts, gay men who are parenting can find themselves in extraordinary demand to share experience and advice and to offer support to others. Some options for gay men to become parents include the following.

As a known donor for lesbians

Acting as a known donor can happen sometimes in a direct relationship with the lesbian or lesbian couple, sometimes again through a third party. It is important that the roles are clearly negotiated and that all parties are comfortable with them. This would not be suitable for a man wanting to be an equal parent, where the request is for an 'arms' length' or 'when the child requests it' known donor. Neither would it suit someone not wanting to be identified as a parent (who may still want to be an anonymous sperm donor). It is also important for each person to indicate the degree of flexibility they will consider. A number of such arrangements we know of have changed after the birth of the child or because of unforeseen circumstances. Systems need to be in place to facilitate future negotiations or changes. Gay male couples may choose to mix their sperm when donating as an act symbolic of their own union.

In partnership as a parent with lesbians or heterosexual women friends
Some gay men and lesbians are choosing to have children together as equal parents, sometimes living in the same household with independent personal lives. Much more rarely gay men may co-parent with heterosexual women friends. These rely on close trusting relationships between the parents, who need clear and shared value systems. Clear ground rules about child care, partners, money, geography, extended family, time and commitment will all help unconventional families to navigate uncharted waters. Sophisticated skills of communication and negotiation will be advantageous as, once more, will wider support networks.

With sole care of children
Some children born as a result of heterosexual unions are cared for solely by a gay man or a gay male couple. It is possible in the future that some lesbians may be prepared to 'donate' children to trusted gay male friends to parent.

Adoption and fostering

A possible route to parenthood is by adoption or fostering. Vetting procedures for prospective parents are stringent and can be discriminatory. Much depends upon the policies of the local authority. Some will consider lesbians and gay men while many will not. At the time of writing the Children's Society, for example, is publicly defending its discrimination against gay prospective parents as being 'in the interests of children'.

Some lesbians present as single women in order to be considered. Some have adopted from other countries, which is a long and stressful process. Children available for adoption or needing foster homes have already experienced upheaval and suffered separation. Difficulties coping with the stresses of this, or of the long uncertain wait, or of the needs of a child from another culture, all might be problems brought to counselling.

There are very few babies available for adoption in Britain for well documented reasons, and these will be placed according to the need of the child. Depending on geography, taking on older children or children with special needs is possible. Some authorities match gay teenagers to gay foster parents. The purpose is the provision of 'good role models'; to be considered one would have to conform to the authority's idea of such a person. The Albert Kennedy Trust is an independent lesbian and gay charity which also offers such a service (see Appendix 2).

Non-parental child care and childlessness

Large numbers of lesbians and gay men are actively involved in child care without themselves being parents. Their contribution to the health, happiness and security of our children is invaluable. It is not, of course, necessary to have a biological connection in order for lesbians and gay men to have mutually rewarding relationships with children. Plenty of children could use another caring adult in their lives, or another role model for maleness and femaleness or for what it means to be adult.

It still remains the case that the majority of lesbians and gay men are childless. This is in itself an identity issue which will present overtly or covertly in the therapy. The language and imagery of childlessness is revealing: fruitless, heirless, barren, sterile, issueless, wasteful, unnatural. Being childless is equated with wasted potential and lack of fulfilment of what's 'natural'. Therapists need to explore their own assumptions about procreation as natural, ordinary, inevitable. These stereotypical prejudices are not far beneath the surface.

The birth families of many childless lesbians and gay men can give messages to them which engender feelings of guilt or inadequacy or even suggest they are cruel for not contributing children to the wider family, without acknowledging the gay person's own feelings at all. It is unsurprising, then, that coming to terms with childlessness will be a difficult and challenging process for many clients, and one in which many will need to deconstruct profound defence or denial systems. Gay men may have found particular difficulty in expressing grief or in having it taken seriously by others.

Against the culturally negative backdrop, the therapist can contextualize the childlessness of the individual and respond appropriately. Has it been consciously chosen by someone who realistically had, or has, the option to have a child? Is the client of a generation for whom having children really was not an option? Is the client someone with HIV or AIDS? In each of these instances, clearly the grieving process will be different. For some it will be the grief of making choices which inevitably close doors, as is true for all of us all the time. 'If I have this, I cannot have that', 'If I do this, I lose that'. For others, it may be the more profoundly personal grief of not having been able to do something which they would very much like to have done. It can be a liberating exploration of ways to be fundamentally creative other than being a parent. For others it could be a key issue to resolve in the preparation for death.

Despite sometimes terrible discrimination, many lesbians and gay men have found, and created, a multitude of ways in which they contribute positively to the lives of children and have gained for themselves many of the rewards for so doing.

Conclusions

- Acknowledging that lesbians and gay men (and to some extent bisexuals putting their same sex passions to the fore) have issues particular to themselves in relation to parenting and not parenting, this chapter has focused a good deal on cultural contexts in which parenting and making families take place. We have described some of the prejudices and discriminations which surround clients and how these can contribute to internalized negative beliefs and feelings.
- All lesbians and gay men have feelings about children, parenting and childlessness and many will have, and more want to have, children of their own. We have looked at some of the ways that this can happen and examined strategies as well as obstacles.
- It is imperative that therapists deconstruct their own belief systems about lesbians, gay men and bisexuals caring for children. They have a valuable role to play, especially in supporting non-traditional families through affirmative therapy, advocacy and educational work with other professionals.
- Lesbian, gay and bisexual parents are justifiably wary of 'child experts' – doctors, social workers, and educationists as well as psychologists and therapists – whose traditionally negative ideas have obstructed these groups parenting. The legal system and the media have made gay parenting extremely precarious, although no evidence exists to endorse beliefs that such families will deprive or harm children or 'make' them homosexual.
- Many lesbian, gay and bisexual people who do not have children continue to make a massive positive contribution to the welfare of society's young.

8 | DOMINIC DAVIES

Working with young people

This chapter aims to help therapists better understand lesbian, gay and bisexual young people and will discuss some specific directives for working with homosexually oriented youth. The reader is also directed to Chapter 4 on coming out for information on what is often the central presenting issue.

Adolescence in our society is often seen as a time of great emotional upheaval, especially with regard to sex and sexuality. In this chapter, I aim not to paint a negative picture of 'troubled times ahead', but also to show some of the positive aspects and issues for young people.

There are a number of things that need to be made clear: first as usual, some definitions. Because a large percentage of adolescents have sexual experiences with others of the same sex, yet only about 5–10 per cent will continue during adulthood to self-identify as gay, it seems important to remind the reader of the differences between:

> *sexual orientation:* 'a preponderance of sexual or erotic feelings, thoughts, fantasies, and/or behaviours ... It is present from an early age – perhaps at conception'.
> (Savin-Williams 1990: 3)

> *sexual identity:* 'a consistent, enduring self-recognition of the meanings that sexual orientation and sexual behaviour have for oneself'.
> (Savin-Williams 1990: 3)

One of the most recent substantive research projects in this area was conducted by Savin-Williams (1990) where a more detailed discussion of prevalence can be found, and from which the following five important findings are taken. All quotations from young people in this chapter are from Burbidge and Walters' important collection of interviews with lesbian and gay teenagers (1981).

Not all homosexual adolescents are sexually active. Boxer (1988) found 9 per cent of boys and 6 per cent of girls self-labelled as gay or lesbian before sexual experiences with the same sex. Manosevitz (1970) found 22 per cent of his sample were 'male homosexual virgins' and Hedblom (1973) found 66 per cent of the female sample were homosexual virgins.

> I've never had sex with a girl before but I have been to bed with a boy once, and that just didn't seem right. If I see a girl I fancy, I'm too scared to approach her, even if I know she is gay.
> (Julie, aged 16; Burbidge and Walters 1981: 18)

Many homosexual adolescents are heterosexually active. Bell and Weinberg (1978) reported that 78 per cent and 79.5 per cent of their sample of gay men and lesbians respectively, had been sexually aroused by a member of the opposite sex.

Many heterosexual adolescents are homosexually active. Figures for men vary between 20 and over 30 per cent (Fay *et al.* 1989; Ramsey 1973) and for women between 5 per cent and 10 per cent (Kinsey *et al.* 1953; Goode and Haber 1977).

> 'Can I ask you something?' said Chris as I got dressed, 'Are you homosexual?'
> It was not a question I had been confronted with before, in spite of having a couple of regular sexual experiences with other boys. 'Yes, I suppose so.'
> 'Yeah, well I'm not,' was the reply.
> Chris and I remained sexual partners, and even teenage lovers for more than three years.
> (Steven, aged 21; Burbidge and Walters 1981: 27)

Many of these issues evoke great stress and anxiety for adolescents of all sexual orientations.

For probably a great many people, their sexuality is not fixed and may change over time. People may change their identity label to coincide with their sexual behaviour, or they may retain a more comfortable identity label. Furthermore, Ross-Reynolds (1982: 70) states:

> The majority of adolescents who engage in homosexual behaviour do not continue this practice into adulthood. Conversely, as many as 31 per cent of gay adults engaged in no homosexual behaviour until they were out of high school.

This information then sets the context for our understanding of lesbian, gay and bisexual youth. Many young people will be having sex with their own gender, but may define themselves as either hetero-, homo- or bisexual, and this may have little bearing on how they self-identify later in life. Some young people with no same sexual experience will still identify as lesbian, gay or bisexual.

Finally, it is important for the reader to remember that most of the research into lesbian, gay and bisexual youth (as with most other research), stems from studies conducted with clinical populations. This is likely to give a biased and problematized view of the experience of being young and gay. It is of course important to remember that this is not the whole picture and that the majority of these young people pass without undue incident into well-adjusted adulthood.

Age of consent

The legal age of consent for male homosexual relations in Great Britain was reduced by the Criminal Justice Act (1994) from 21 to 18 years old. This came about after an intensive campaign of lobbying and political action initiated by the gay community, with the intention of lowering the age of consent to 16 to bring about parity with heterosexual sexual consent. In spite of august bodies such as the British Medical Association and the National Children's Bureau supporting the case for equality, the motion for a common age of consent of 16 fell by 28 votes.

It is highly unlikely that the differential age of consent is going to deter young people from having sex; what it does do is contribute immeasurably to the low self-esteem of young people, and obstruct service providers from actively supporting and helping them.

There has been little formal research conducted into the effects on the mental and sexual health of young people of knowing they are having sex under the legal age of consent. Coyle (1994) points to the stresses young gay men experience when we consider that in his survey of 151 gay men, the mean age of 'self-suspicion' was 14 years, but that self-definition didn't occur until almost six years later (19.8 years), with the mean age for coming out to someone else being 21.6 years. Coyle (1994: 3) goes on:

> Respondents in the study of gay identity formation frequently said they experienced fear (51.1 per cent) and isolation (48.2 per cent) at this point [their teens]. Many said they knew they didn't fit the stereotype of the effeminate gay man (48.2 per cent) and they didn't know what to do next (47.5 per cent). Their suspicions about their sexuality also affected their social behaviour. Many thought they would have to be very secretive (71.1 per cent) and became very concerned about what other people thought of them (71.1 per cent).

We could easily speculate how knowledge that one is a sex criminal might affect how easily young men feel able to approach official agencies for support. If a 16-year-old gay man became infected with a sexually transmitted disease, how comfortable might he be approaching his GP? If he became depressed over the ending of a relationship, how likely would he be to approach a local authority youth worker? Legally he would be 'confessing' to a crime. The fact that most workers would (hopefully) ignore the legality of the issue and offer help is irrelevant if young people are *deterred* from approaching services for support.

We should also reflect on the effect of being a sex criminal on the self-esteem of the young person. Since society imposes an unequal age of consent for gay male sexual relations, what impact might this have on the young person's feeling of self-worth? What implications might this have for those charged with educating young people about HIV/AIDS? How might this affect the work of teachers in school trying to prevent anti-gay bullying? This change in the law will almost undoubtedly reinforce feelings of being second class citizens for lesbian, gay and bisexual young people.

Hetrick and Martin (1987) have identified isolation as the most critical issue affecting most lesbian, gay and bisexual young people. From their pioneering work at Hetrick-Martin Institute (formerly the Institute for the Protection of Lesbian and Gay Youth), which they founded in New York in 1979, they found three key areas where isolation served to detrimentally affect the lives of the young: these were social, emotional and cognitive.

Social isolation

Feeling isolated from their peers, many lesbian, gay and bisexual young people will withdraw from socializing because the situation may raise difficult feelings. Socializing with the same sex may awaken strong sexual or emotional feelings, and socializing with the other sex may remind them of the absence of any heterosexual interest and difference from their heterosexual peers. Rivers's (1994, 1995a) research shows that many young people are isolated and bullied because of their actual or perceived homosexuality.

There are still very few lesbian and gay youth groups in Britain. The few that do exist are often poorly resourced. Local education authority funding and support is the exception rather than the rule, particularly in the light of Section 28 of the Local Government Act 1988, which sought to prevent local authorities from 'intentionally promoting homosexuality'.

Lesbian and gay youth groups have a history of being peer led, rather than having trained youth workers employed to support the membership. Whilst the reasons for this are generally economic, the result is that at best they can be excellent models of self-empowerment, and at worst they may be quite difficult and stressful places for an already isolated lesbian or gay young person to go along to.

It is suggested that therapists check out the existence and nature of their local group before referring a young person to it. It is also helpful to remember that this picture may change regularly, as the membership may move on to other things.

Hetrick and Martin (1987) also observed that social isolation can lead to young gay men finding places where they can meet others for sexual contact, but where social interaction is difficult, for example through cottaging (meeting others for sex in public toilets). This can create a pattern where sex is the initial stage of social interaction rather than a behaviour stemming from connection on other levels. It can also contribute to a young person's sense of low self-esteem, whereby he feels people only want to have sex with him, and this may confirm internalized negative messages about the promiscuity of gay men. There can, of course, be other dangers – to the young person's health and safety. For their adult male partners, the current legal situation, which prohibits sex with men under the age of 18, means that a more complete relationship may be too risky.

For young lesbians, their social isolation can mean that when they do meet another lesbian, they may become locked into a 'merged' relationship which obstructs the opportunity to develop other friendships (see Chapter 6). Rothblum (1990) argues that the isolation of young lesbians promotes depression, substance abuse and self-destructive behaviour.

Emotional isolation

This may be apparent in feeling emotionally withdrawn from their families, the need to hide their sexuality and be on their guard at all times. Young people may feel betrayed by their emotions because of their homosexual desires, and try to shut down on any kind of emotional life. Depression is an obvious result of this, and research has shown that 20 per cent of lesbian and gay young people attempt suicide (Trenchard and Warren 1984; Hetrick and Martin 1987). Ian Rivers's interesting work at the University of Luton suggests that bullying and other reinforcements of homophobia promote social and emotional withdrawal, isolation and depression in later life. Additionally, the absence of support from peers and fear of disclosure to parents and teachers and subsequent rejection, further promote feelings of hopelessness and despair, leading to thoughts of self-harm or suicide. He cites a 1989 US Department of Health and Human Services Task Force on Suicide report that lesbian and gay youths were five times more likely to attempt suicide than their heterosexual peers (see Rivers 1994, 1995a, 1995b).

Cognitive isolation

There is an almost complete absence of accurate information about homosexuality available to young people. School libraries are often too afraid of holding positive books about homosexuality, and even where such books are held, because of the social stigma attached to homosexuality, the young person may be afraid to take the books out. The absence of appropriate role models means that young people often believe the most appalling stereotypes because that is all that is available to them. This may lead them to believe that they have to act out some of these stereotypes themselves, or to continue to deny their sexuality and prolong their isolation and delay coming to terms with their homosexuality. More extensive discussion of homophobia and the process of 'coming out' is to be found in Chapters 3 and 4.

Case example 1
One example of this isolation manifesting itself is demonstrated by Jamie, a 15-year-old gay man, referred to his school counsellor because he was being bullied at school. He arrived at his first appointment wearing make-up and feminine clothing. His effeminate manner had resulted in him becoming socially ostracized by his male peers. He told the counsellor he had known he was gay since he was 9. Just recently he'd started to hang out with a bunch of drag queens at the local gay pub. He felt society expected him to behave like a woman, since he wasn't 'a real man' and that by cross-dressing he was challenging people. Those people who could accept his behaviour demonstrated acceptance of Jamie. He was very lonely. The counsellor helped Jamie see that he was still male and there were things he still enjoyed about being male, so that there was no need for him to become a camp stereotype in order to be gay. His cross-dressing was a provocative behaviour unconsciously designed to bring about rejection, since he felt unwanted, except by the drag queens. Through meeting a broader range of lesbian and gay people, and after some supportive work with his counsellor on his self-esteem, Jamie felt able to drop the effeminate façade at school and saved his 'dragging up' for situations where it was more appropriate.

Self-esteem issues

This isolation will almost inevitably affect the young person's feelings of self-worth. Internalized homophobia can affect young people in a variety of ways, I will focus here on three key areas: HIV/AIDS, suicide, and sexual abuse.

HIV/AIDS

If a gay or bisexual young man feels bad about his sexuality, then it is possible he will fail to protect himself when having sex. Lack of self-confidence may lead to his not being assertive in negotiating safer sex. He may not feel his life is worth protecting, since he sees a future of discrimination and ridicule. He may be meeting partners for sex whilst intoxicated by alcohol or other drugs, and his resistance to having safer sex may therefore be lowered. Some research from Australia has shown that people are more likely to follow safer sex messages when they feel involved in the gay community:

> In general, men in contact with others, via attachment to gay community – sexual, social or cultural/political – are most likely to have changed their sexual practice. They have the informed social support necessary to modify their behaviour. Men who are isolated from others like themselves and are unattached to gay community in any form are those least likely to change.
> (Kippax et al. 1992: 116)

This research raises important implications for the education of young people about safer sex and, more importantly perhaps, maintaining safer sex behaviour. Young people new to coming out, feeling isolated, and not having yet had much chance to challenge the myths and stereotypes about homosexuality are not best placed to feel an integral part of the gay community or to feel self-esteem adequate to make their own health and well-being a priority.

Therapists can have an important role here in helping clients to explore feelings about HIV and safer sex, and the reader's attention is drawn to the work of Shernoff (1989) who believes that therapists are ideally placed to help clients explore this sensitive area, providing we are comfortable in speaking explicitly about sexual matters and are informed about HIV and safer sex issues. This was referred to in greater depth in Chapter 2.

Suicide/parasuicide

Several studies, including a British one (Trenchard and Warren 1984) mentioned above, have found at least 20 per cent of young lesbian, gay and bisexual people have made suicide attempts. Suicide is the second highest cause of death amongst young people. Verdicts of 'misadventure' and 'accidental death' are sometimes returned by coroners, where it is not entirely clear whether a young person killed themselves, to spare the family the shame and guilt still attached to a verdict of suicide. It is impossible to estimate how many young people each year do succeed in killing themselves because of the difficulties they experience and foresee in living their life as lesbian, gay or bisexual, but the figures are probably quite high.

Since sexual orientation seems to be beyond our active control, like our eye colour, it is a sad indictment of our society that people are driven to kill themselves because they cannot see a future as lesbian, gay and bisexual people. It would be nonsensical for someone to kill themselves because they had blue eyes, yet every year young people take their lives because they cannot bear the thought of living with a stigmatized identity.

Sexual abuse

Martin and Hetrick (1987) found incidence of 22 per cent of the young people presenting to their project reported being sexually abused. This figure is probably an underestimate, since many young people do not present with sexual abuse, but may raise it later on, when they feel safer in their counselling. The abuse of young lesbians and gay men is often by members of their family (an uncle, or older brother, sometimes a father). It is common for young victims to blame themselves for the abuse, believing that it occurred because of their homosexual desire. Other young people may believe that their homosexuality results *from* having been sexually abused. Research does not support this 'causal' link, but it reflects their belief in being damaged by the abuse, and now having to live with a 'damaged' sexuality. Young lesbians may be sexually abused as a way of punishing them for their homosexuality and to reinforce male power and control.

Young lesbians and gay men are vulnerable to sexual exploitation by older people because of their isolation. Martin and Hetrick found that when young people were given the opportunity to mix with their peers, then they often felt able to move out of any exploitative relationship they may have had with older people.

The lesbian and gay community response

Many adult lesbians or gay men are afraid to get involved in supporting lesbian and gay youth because of the fears of being suspected of sexual motives or even accused of sexual abuse due to societal links between homosexuality and paedophilia. This is despite large numbers of lesbian, gay and bisexual people working in youth service agencies.

> Whether due to inadequate professional knowledge, fear of jeopardising professional positions, or simple lack of interest, personnel in youth-serving agencies and school districts (many of whom are gay themselves) have for the most part, not been willing to speak out on behalf of gay youth.
>
> (Robinson 1984: 14)

This results in increasing the isolation and alienation experienced by the young.

Isolated from well-functioning gay or lesbian adult role models by lack of access and fears of reprisal, young gay men and lesbians frequently resort to bars, or public meeting places where they are apt to meet persons who are intoxicated, marginally functional, and emotionally or sexually exploitative.

(Gonsiorek 1988: 116)

One of the positive aspects to draw attention to here is that there are many lesbian and gay adults who do spend a great deal of their time and energy, usually as volunteers on gay helplines, supporting the young. Their contribution to the developing identities of lesbian, gay and bisexual young people is immense.

Because of the paucity of gay affirmative youth services and the lack of social and community provision which is not commercially centred around alcohol, many young people wanting to be with others for social support are forced to do so in gay pubs and clubs. The easy access to alcohol and recreational drug use can mean them self-medicating to ease the pressures of being in a stigmatized minority, or else be seen as a necessary adjunct to inclusion in a group.

It might be helpful for the reader to be reminded of Grace's (1977) concept of 'developmental lag' highlighted by Coleman (1981/82) and referred to in Chapter 4, when considering the support of adult lesbians, gay men and bisexuals for their younger 'kin'. The lag can be helpful when older people, still working out some of their own developmental tasks from adolescence, find it quite easy to relate to, and be supportive of, younger people. Differences in chronological age may create difficulties in other areas as some adults might be 'stuck' in their developmental process and *only* attracted to young people, and this may be experienced in a predatory way by the young person concerned. I think this is what Gonsiorek meant by his use of the phrase 'marginally functional, and emotionally or sexually exploitative' (Gonsiorek 1988: 116).

School and education issues

School is obviously a central part of a young person's life. Most of the waking day for those aged between 5 to 16 years old, and for an increasing minority even older, is spent within educational institutions. For the young lesbian, gay or bisexual person, these institutions can be appalling places. I have already looked at the isolation experienced by the young lesbian, gay and bisexual person. To this picture I should now add physical and verbal harassment. Bullying is extremely common in most of our schools (Rivers 1995a). The most common taunts are 'poof', 'queer' and 'lezzie'. Of course these taunts are not limited to homosexually oriented young people. Probably most young people who get bullied will get called these names. However, for those that aren't lesbian, gay or bisexual, the taunt will be meaningless – empty words. For the homosexually oriented young person, the jeer may well represent a more sinister attack on their self-esteem: 'How can they know this about me?' 'What signal am I giving off?'

The bullying may then cause the young person to withdraw socially, to concentrate on their studies, to align themselves with school life and the system; in some schools this may be schools council or becoming a prefect. Other young people may start to drop out of school prematurely, some will (through the process of reaction formation) become bullies and develop a hypermasculine tough guy approach. Whichever way the young person copes with the harassment, their psychosocial development is likely to be impaired as is their level of educational achievement or sense of fulfilment with what is achieved.

It is our contention in this book that the pathologizing, and even criminalizing, of something as central to selfhood as one's sexuality, is necessarily injurious to the young. The cultural climate created by such processes also provides a framework for bullying and isolation during crucial phases of identity formation.

The invisibility of homosexuality in the curriculum is another factor which can isolate the lesbian, gay and bisexual young person. The fact that many of the people studied in literature, science, music, art, etc. were homosexual, and that homosexuality informed their work, is usually omitted from the teaching about them.

Teachers who are willing to provide non-biased information about homosexuality, including referrals to gay affirmative reading and support agencies, can make a tremendous difference to the lives of young people concerned about their sexuality:

> People at school know and a few tease me. They say 'Get lost, you queer' and make other nasty comments. I told a teacher that I was depressed and that I was a lesbian. She was very liberal and thought it fantastic that I could tell her. She didn't say anything about it being 'a phase'.
>
> (Elizabeth, 15 years; Burbidge and Walters 1981: 10–11)

Those helpers working in education may find Epstein (1994) and Harris (1990) helpful.

Work and employment issues

Whether we are considering employment training or paid work, as with school, should the young person not hide their sexuality the potential for harassment is great. This may be more acute for young men than for women, and is more likely to take the form of physical and verbal intimidation, usually by other males. The openly gay or bisexual man seems to act as a threat to a hypermasculine ideal. Young lesbians, unless they have a gender atypical appearance, are likely to be presumed heterosexual and heterosexist assumptions serve to make their sexuality invisible. The young dyke with a shaved head and Doc Martin boots is probably just as likely to be intimidated as the openly gay or bisexual young man.

Unemployment or low paid 'employment training' serves to keep young people economically dependent on their parents. This has an additional psychosocial significance for lesbian, gay and bisexual young persons in that it holds them captive in a suspended adolescence. If their parents are unsympathetic to their homosexuality, opportunities for achieving other social and emotional developmental tasks of adolescence may be held up. Some young women and men never leave home; remaining unmarried often means they are expected to live at home and later care for aged parents.

Occupational choice and the lesbian, gay and bisexual adolescent

Many adolescents seek work in which they are intellectually underachieving, and where this includes a sympathetic response to their homosexuality they prefer to remain in it. There are a number of low paid areas of work which have been traditionally sympathetic to employing lesbians and gay men. For men these would include some service industries (clothes shops, floristry, hairdressing, nursing) and the field of entertainment. For lesbians, service industries again predominate and would include bar work, sports coaching, and some manual trades. A fairly large proportion of lesbians and gay men seek work within the police force and the armed forces, environments which have generally been actively hostile. This may be changing since some police forces have now included sexual orientation in their equal opportunities policies and are trying to develop a service which more accurately reflects the communities they serve (for a detailed account of life for lesbians, gay men and bisexuals in the police see Burke 1993). The Criminal Justice Act 1994 decriminalized homosexual sexual acts between consenting men in the armed forces, although it has done nothing to lift the ban on *being* gay and lesbians and gay men can still be dismissed because of their sexuality regardless of their conduct. The military authorities have attempted to maintain powers to dismiss those *open* about their homosexuality from the forces. Four sacked officers, backed by the lobby group, Stonewall, have been challenging discrimination of this kind in the British courts. These test cases, attracting a number of sympathetic judgements along the way, will undoubtedly bring about a change in the law.

Work with young people – particularly teaching, youth work and social work – attracts a high proportion of lesbian, gay and bisexual people to make their careers. However these choices may be precarious for people who choose not to hide their sexuality. It is not uncommon for lesbians, gay men and bisexuals to lose their jobs or to be ignored for promotion because of answering questions or being open about their sexuality. The myths that young people are at risk of seduction, and that homosexuality is intrinsically attractive to young people create a tension which almost certainly impairs the worker's ability to do their job properly, since they are having to hide a vital aspect of themselves. Not being able to be open means they are also unable to provide positive role models of the diversity of lesbians, gay men and bisexuals in society, thus contributing further to the internalized self-oppression and shame of the young gay people, and further to the unchallenged prejudice of homophobic youngsters, with whom they are working.

Working in business and commerce, where there is often an expectation of home entertaining or attending business functions accompanied by a spouse, can create anxiety for many people in same sex relationships. Sometimes people in such situations will seek the support of friends of the other sex to act as escorts. This 'passing' can further damage self-esteem by compounding internalized homophobia.

Parents and family issues

Many young people hold an ambivalent position with regard to coming out to their families. Some strongly deny wanting their parents to know, yet will leave gay newspapers and books around their rooms, and even open diaries by their bedside. It would take a self-restraint of iron not to notice these things. This unconscious longing is not too surprising when, to maintain ego integrity, one has to manage the tension between knowing one will be popularly viewed as mad, bad and dangerous to know, and needing support and affirmation from the people one is closest to.

The lesbian, gay and bisexual young person is more likely to tell a sibling before telling their parents. Trenchard and Warren (1984) found just over 8 per cent of their sample came out to a sibling first, whereas 7.5 per cent came out to their mother first and 0.6 per cent (two young men) came out to their fathers first. Parental reactions vary. Often when parents react badly, the young person may get a positive reaction from another sibling.

> Just after I left school, with no friends at all, I got depressed one evening and told Dorian (my older brother) about my gay feelings. He seemed to understand completely and he told me that everyone goes through life fancying both sexes, to one extent or another ... He told

me that I wasn't sick and that I shouldn't be ashamed of finding girls attractive.

[on telling her mother] ... as I told her, she burst into tears and called the doctor immediately. I couldn't help laughing, because everything was so helpless and ridiculous. I'll have to move to another area now, because my mother just won't speak to me any more and Dad says the sooner I leave, the better. He says 'No daughter of mine is going to bring my name into disrepute'.

(Lorraine, aged 17; Burbidge and Walters 1981: 37)

There is evidence to suggest (Holtzen and Agresti 1990) that those parents who are most homophobic are ones who hold traditional beliefs about how men and women should behave, have a lower sense of social self-esteem, and have known about their child's lesbian or gay identity for a relatively short period of time (under two years). Of course this is not always the case, as Steven's experience reflects:

my parents even to this day will not talk about gayness unless forced to, and will not have a picture of myself and my boyfriend on their mantelpiece or even in a bedroom, and they've known my present lover for three and a half years. Things like that are small, but do hurt.

(Steven, aged 21; Burbidge and Walters 1981: 28)

Parents may also seek help from counsellors and therapists. Sometimes this is as a result of discovering their child is lesbian, gay or bisexual and they metaphorically (although sometimes literally) drag their offspring along by their ear, and demand that the therapist 'cure' them of the homosexuality. It is possible for inexperienced therapists to deride such parents and think only of providing direct support and sympathy to the young person concerned. This view is unwise for two reasons: unhappy parents will result in more stress for the young person and unhappy parents will result in unhappy parents! Both parties are entitled to help and support. Bernstein (1990) found five major themes emerging in her work with parents of lesbian and gay young people: social stigma; self- and/or spouse-blame; parental losses; fears and concerns for the gay child; and fear of losing their son or daughter if they did not accept the child's homosexuality. Much work can be done with parents directly, through recommended reading and through referral to self-help support organizations such as Family and Friends of Lesbians and Gays (FFLAG) (see Appendix 2). Research has further shown that in order to change homophobic attitudes one needs to address both the cognitive and affective elements and clearly well informed therapists play an important part in this process.

Cramer and Roach (1988) found, in their survey of attitudes of parents to their son's coming out as gay, that parents with strong 'traditional' values do appear to change their views when their own son is involved. On the other hand, the son who expects his liberal and non-homophobic parents to respond immediately in a positive way to his disclosure may be disappointed since most parents seem to have difficulty with immediate acceptance. However, given time, most families come to accept their son's homosexuality.

Cramer and Roach's research was done with white, middle-class, college-educated American males and the data should not automatically be extrapolated to women, people of colour or those from the working class, whose experiences may be quite different. Also 'acceptance' does not describe measures of affirmation or celebration.

Caught with their trousers down

When parents seek therapy for children under 14 whom they have caught experimenting sexually with a same sex friend, it is likely that they will attach far more significance to such activity amongst peers than would the young person themselves. The parents may overreact and be angry, hurt and disgusted. They may demand that the therapist 'cure' the child's homosexuality.

Woodman and Lenna (1980) suggest that in such circumstances the therapist initially sees the parents alone. Whilst they are likely to want to talk about the 'act', the therapist's role is to explore how the discovery has affected the relationship between parents and child and to get a picture of previous family dynamics. The aim of the therapy is to try to restore the family to its previous level of interaction, or perhaps to increase their ability to respond in a loving and supportive way.

Woodman and Lenna suggest therapists help parents understand that homosexual activity, particularly in preadolescent years, is not necessarily indicative of a lesbian or gay orientation. Sexual experimentation does not have the same motivation or significance for children that it does for adults. It is important to remind them that pre-teen children are likely to believe what their parents say as absolute and if the parents say the child is sick, evil or queer, the child is likely to believe them and internalize these negative messages with damaging long term consequences, especially should the child develop same sex preferences.

It is important to re-establish positive family relations. The same sex parent should be encouraged to show affection, and other family members, if they become involved in the 'crisis', should also be helped to affirm and support the child. The child should continue to be allowed to play with same sex friends, including those involved in the sexual experimentation.

Woodman and Lenna then suggest seeing the child. The counsellor has two goals here: to express that sex is not a bad thing and that parents often see sex as belonging to the adult world and second, to acknowledge that the parents may have said things which hurt and upset the child, because they were surprised and upset themselves. It is important to reassure the child of the parents' love, which they may feel is lost.

The same approach can be helpful with young people over 14. Parents and therapists should not attach more significance to same sex activity than the young person concerned. It is important to remember that Kinsey *et al.* (1947) found that 60 per cent of their total male sample engaged in some form of homosexual behaviour before 16 and, for a quarter of them, this behaviour was on more than a few occasions. These figures are much higher than the generally accepted 10 per cent of adults who have a consistent lesbian or gay orientation and so premature labelling is unhelpful.

For the 10 per cent (and it is likely to be higher in under 21-year-olds), it is important that they have an affirming and understanding response with access to as much information about, and support for, their developing sexuality as they want.

Conflict with the family and the role of social services

It is common for lesbian and gay young people to be rejected and mistreated by their families. Trenchard and Warren (1984) found that 21 per cent of British lesbian and gay young people reported being beaten up because of their homosexuality and 11 per cent were thrown out of their homes. Should the family come to the attention of social work agencies, then the young person often becomes pathologized as the focus of the family's dysfunction – 'the identified patient'.

If the young person is placed into local authority care (as sometimes happens when parents reject their children's sexuality), residential social workers, used to dealing with disturbed teenagers, can be overwhelmed by a comparatively well-adjusted, well-behaved lesbian, gay or bisexual young person, especially if they are non-white, gender atypical and working class. Being placed in local authority care feels like being punished for being gay and the young person may understandably feel outrage, fear, distress or hatred. They are likely to meet a number of highly disturbed young people, and possibly be introduced to dysfunctional coping strategies including solvent abuse, deliberate self-harm, unsafe promiscuity or criminal behaviours. It is not unknown in such establishments (particularly for male staff, where there is a high value placed on machismo and hypermasculinity) to collude with or even provoke bullying, including physical violence towards young people placed in their care.

Often sexual orientation becomes the focus of 'treatment', rather than other more relevant issues (for example, the young person's safety, housing, and access to peer support, their feelings and needs). Well-intentioned staff may lack adequate information, resources and training to help them respond appropriately.

It is the author's view that there are very few circumstances which can justify a lesbian, gay or bisexual young person being placed into residential care. There are nearly always alternatives; staying with the family of a sympathetic friend, foster care with foster parents experienced in such situations; or placement with carers registered with the Albert Kennedy Trust (see Appendix 2) are acceptable avenues. The potential damage to a young person's self-esteem following a parental rejection is such that residential care is likely to compound the problem, rather than provide any kind of 'safe haven'.

Guidelines for therapists working with lesbian, gay and bisexual youth

Therapists need to remember that they should be supporting the autonomy and empowerment of their clients, however young. This may mean a need to be vigilant over their counter-transference and not to get caught up in the role of parenting the young person. For some workers who may be working officially in *loco parentis* there may be difficulties around being able to offer complete confidentiality; they should be open with their client about the limitations of confidentiality *before* the young person reveals their material.

When working with young people, therapists should:

- respect the young person's feelings, experiences, and integrity;
- offer time and space to help the young person explore and reflect upon their experiences and feelings;
- offer suggestions of reading material (see Appendix 3) and information about youth groups, gay helping agencies and other resources (see Appendix 2);
- be sure to locate the problem as homophobia and not the client's homosexuality;
- be willing to offer information (possibly again in written form) and education about sexual matters and to discuss HIV awareness, possibly through role playing negotiating skills;
- find ways of enhancing self-esteem.

When working with the family of a lesbian, gay or bisexual young person, therapists should:

- ensure they support the young person by maintaining confidentiality;
- with permission, act as advocate for the young person by helping the parent to understand homosexuality better (again written information may be helpful here);

- help the parents work through their own homophobia, gender stereotyping and expectations. (Their son coming out as gay does not seek to undermine the masculinity of the father. Likewise, the daughter's lesbianism is not an attack on the mother's femininity. Neither reflects in any way on their parenting);
- reassure parents that their child's sexuality was not a result of anything they did or didn't do, are, or are not;
- offer accurate, non-technical information about homosexuality and introductions to parent support groups such as FFLAG (mentioned earlier);
- acknowledge, affirm and work through each family member's own feelings about the child's gayness to facilitate mutual understanding.

The therapist's role within society is:

- to be an advocate for lesbian, gay and bisexual youth, representing and speaking up for them where they may not feel able to speak out for themselves, and challenge the homophobia and heterosexism which causes them suffering;
- to offer workshops and training for colleagues to provide opportunities to discuss, and if necessary, challenge, some of the myths and stereotypes about homosexuality;
- to offer consultancy within their institution to heads, governors, etc. on how to ensure the environment can become a safer, more affirming place in which all young people can develop and integrate their sexuality without harm;
- to be prepared within personal and professional groups and in wider society to support equalities issues.

Conclusions

- Adolescence can be a stressful and anxious time in western society and emergent sexual identity will be a key factor.
- Young people who have sex with their own gender may or may not identify as lesbian, gay or bisexual then or later.
- Those who do may encounter verbal, physical or sexual abuse in the family homes, at school, in the work place or in local authority residential care.
- The continued criminalization of one sexual orientation – male homosexuality – has profound implications for mental health, self-esteem, bullying, isolation, lack of advice and guidance, unsafe sexual behaviours, suicide, self-harm, HIV and AIDS.
- Many adult lesbians, gay men and bisexuals do devote time and energy to supporting young members of these communities, while many others

are afraid to do so due to societal connection of homosexuality and paedophilia.
- Research reveals that schooling, the central activity of young lives, can be a hostile and damaging experience for bisexual and homosexual youth, causing some to withdraw from peers and others to leave education early and insufficiently qualified or motivated to go further.
- Lesbian, gay and bisexual adolescents are equally likely to settle for low paid, undemanding employment in environments less hostile to their sexuality or in jobs such as child care, the police or military where they have to conceal their true identity.
- Parents need support from therapists in working through feelings about stigma, blame and loss and their fears about their child's homosexuality. Other family members need similar support and siblings can be most helpful to the young person concerned.
- Sexual orientation *per se*, or family rejection as a reaction to it, are never acceptable reasons for placement into residential care and social services need to find friends or foster parents who can offer secure, loving alternatives.
- Therapists working with the young need to affirm the ego identity and integrity of the client in helping them explore, express and reflect upon their feelings and experiences, and will have an educative function, too. They will be sure clearly to identify homophobia, not the client's sexuality, as pathological.
- Affirmative therapists have an invaluable role in society as advocates and consultants within a wide range of groups, building a safer environment in which the young can develop identities without being harmed.

9 | VAL YOUNG

Working with older lesbians

This chapter is intended to give context to several possible issues for lesbians in therapy, including specific problems discussed elsewhere. There will, unavoidably in a short chapter, be simplification, generalization and selectivity. Anecdotes are chosen from the author's interviews or widely available publications.

The number of older lesbians is increasing. This is partly due to the ageing population, but it is more relevant to recognize that lesbians of all ages are far more visible now than at any time in British history. The profound political changes since the 1970s have enabled more lesbians, including many who were married to men, to come out. This applies in particular to lesbian members of other differentiated and marginalized groups, who were until recently doubly invisible.

Several lesbian and feminist reappraisals of psychoanalysis and psychology have brought sexuality studies into the forefront of academic debate, and new lesbian professional writings are beginning to influence therapy practice in general.

Who are older lesbians?

There is no simple definition of 'older' and therapy can be made more effective by respecting the historical complexities of women's sexual self-identification. The factors which created these complexities, in themselves frequent therapy issues, can be used as frameworks to simplify the process for both client and practitioner. What is usually described as a client's 'social context' is also, and more accurately, generational – the continual legal and social changes which directly affect lesbians, their personal circumstances, their birth communities and their wider social environments. Chapter 10 discusses some of these issues in relation to older gay men.

The term 'older lesbian' is also a political statement about a collective historical identity. For all lesbians who have come out in the past two decades, it is a challenge to ageist perceptions of women's sexuality, mental health, psychological flexibility, social roles and usefulness to society as a whole. 'Mid-life', 'older', and 'old', while convenient categories for discussing therapy, health, and social issues, cannot be taken as rigid definitions of new 'minority' groups, since most lesbians will choose, or not, such identifications for themselves.

The formation of a lesbian identity

The establishment of separate lesbian and bisexual identities is a twentieth-century western phenomenon (Bland 1983). The first openly lesbian novel, Radclyffe Hall's *The Well of Loneliness*, was banned within weeks of publication in 1928 (in the UK only) because it supported lesbian sexuality and pleaded for public understanding. There were no images of lesbians until its reissue in 1949. Even novels published in the 'swinging sixties', such as Maureen Duffy's mournful study of London life, *The Microcosm* (1967), re-enforced negative stereotypes. The formative years of women over 45 who have lived all their adult years as lesbians 'were spent in the fearful, hidden and self-hating world before the women's movement and gay liberation, and [their] later years are being spent in an era totally revolutionized by these movements' (Sang *et al.* 1991: 3). 'Lifelong' older lesbians, therefore, form a unique population group, one which was previously kept – legally – invisible, except in psychoanalytic or psychiatric textbooks.

It cannot be assumed that all lesbians have benefited from the post-war human rights campaigns, and this patchwork history has particular implications in therapy. Most lesbians also carry a history of other, multiple, oppressions, sexism being the most damaging, and psychotherapy played a major role in reinforcing lesbian stigmatizing during the 1950s. Lesbians were pathologized as 'psychotic' women suffering from gender disorders (Klaich 1974; O'Connor and Ryan 1993; Chodorow 1994).

These distorted views spawned several pop psychology books (for example Caprio 1954) which were fed by and reinforced social, religious and political prejudices. This meant that lesbians either led double lives married to men, but without a chosen bisexual identity were prevented from coming out, or were deprived of opportunities for mothering. Individuals, couples and groups (for instance, those in the armed forces) were isolated from each other until the formation of social networks in the 1960s. Diana Chapman, Esme Langley and three others started the first British lesbian magazine

Arena 3 in 1964; it had come out of the Minorities Research Group and led to a social network. Some members went on to form *Kenric* in 1965 and *Sappho* in 1973. Many had thought they were the only lesbian in the world: 'I felt as if I invented myself', one 55-year-old disabled lesbian wrote (Beckett 1989).

Lesbian oppression is invisible in the formerly 'radical' therapies which, since the early 1990s, have become professional, charitable and 'apolitical' (Young 1995b). While many lesbians may never raise sexuality issues in therapy, well-intentioned equalities policies, such as those that underpin new NVQ standards or codes of ethics, separate lesbians (or bisexual women) from, for instance, black, Asian, disabled, old, or working-class women. There is little recognition that a lesbian can identify with more than one marginalized group. On the contrary, they are invariably grouped collectively as in 'lesbian, gay and bisexual'.

Older lesbians and therapy

Client self-definition and a realistic appraisal of individual needs are essential for any effective therapeutic work. A first step could be the personal meaning of 'older'. When they are grouped together as 'over 50', for example, this is 'another way of disempowering lesbians' (Hemmings 1989).

Practitioners need to take into account both the omission, outside feminism, of affirmative therapy models, and the history of lesbians' social oppression. If, for example, a 'mid-life' transition triggers a renewed search for a positive identity, this can mean re-evaluating the past and exploring long buried traumas. 'I realised a lot of oppression I hadn't dealt with before, because I had never viewed my life as a lesbian before' (Hall Carpenter Archives/Lesbian History Group 1989: 2).

It is reasonable to state that therapy has never viewed lesbians' lives before; analytic theories deal principally with the development of (heterosexual) gender identity and, in combination with traditional pathologizing attitudes, this meant that older lesbians may never have considered therapy as an option or as relevant or accessible to them. A US survey by a lesbian and gay counselling agency in Seattle found that in its first five years, only 1 per cent of its clients were aged 30–60, and no statistics were available for clients older than 60 (Klein 1991: 181).

In the UK, many lesbians were able to find their own means of self-empowerment, including political work. Others opted for feminist or radical therapies or formed self-help groups 'to have a therapy that we can control ourselves' (Ernst and Goodison 1981: 4). It should be added that lesbian self-help also provides security against risks of further professional judgements of problematic issues, such as violence, addictions, psychiatric labels or sexual difficulties, and their appearances in 'case studies' in psychotherapy journals. For example, childhood sexual abuse is frequently believed to be a 'cause' of 'lesbianism' (Bass and Davis 1988: 268):

> A 52-year-old lesbian said: 'I was sexually abused, and all these years I never talked to anyone about it because of what people say. I saw an advert for a lesbian counsellor who worked with sexual abuse. I was on the phone the next day, and I haven't stopped talking since. I'm learning how being abused caused me a lot of problems, but the one thing I'm sure about that is that being a lesbian was never a *problem* for me. It's such a relief to have got this sorted out after 30 years.'

Older lesbians also have been affected by therapy's traditional ageism, which meant that women over 50 were considered 'a poor investment for therapy, too resistant to change, or simply untreatable' (Barnes and Maple 1992: 98).

Resources

The exploration of ageing is relatively new for lesbians, and there are several areas of conflict. There is a frequent assertion that 'most... lesbian elders feel free and comfortable with themselves' and are 'well prepared for ageing, since we are accustomed to being responsible for our own lives' (Hepburn and Gutierrez 1988: 85). Such generalizations obscure the realities of ageing. Said a lesbian whose retirement coincided with the end of a 25 year partnership, 'People assume that I've made it to 60, I've got it all together. I'm a survivor, a wise crone, and all that rubbish'.

The position of lesbians or bisexual women in the psychiatric system has only recently been formally acknowledged, and it was late in 1994 before lesbian (and gay) groups were set up by the mental health charity MIND, which in June 1995 held the first 'lesbian, gay and bisexual' mental health conference (see Appendix 2).

The most reliable sources of information are older lesbians themselves. Recordings of personal histories, including those of older black and Asian lesbians, were begun as a result of the UK's first Older Lesbians Conference in 1984, which founded a self-organized social and support network. One book of oral histories was compiled for a 1991 Channel 4 television film, *Women Like Us*. These are documents of survival, determination, humour and creativity by lesbians up to their late 80s. They offer, though unintentionally, insights to a number of therapy issues and, frequently, solutions (Hall Carpenter Archives/Lesbian History Group 1989; Neild and Pearson 1992). Early in 1994 a funded project for lesbians over the age of 50 was set up by the Association of Greater London Older Women (AGLOW) (see Appendix 2 for details of these organizations).

The wealth of material produced in the USA and Canada offers a valuable resource, although there is more research on lifestyles than on therapy issues. While these texts also expose the comparatively limited options for lesbians living in the UK, they can suggest models for creative approaches to mid-life and ageing which both avoid problem consciousness and offer a deeper philosophy than most therapies provide (Rothblum and Cole 1989; Sang *et al.* 1991; Card 1992; Stevens 1993). Lesbian health guides, Black women's health guides and British editions of women's publications which include lesbian health concerns in a multicultural context remain the best resources for both clients and practitioners (Hepburn and Gutierrez 1988; Phillips and Rakusen 1989; Shapiro 1989). There were, unexpectedly, no references to ageing issues in a recent North American study of psychological perspectives on lesbian and gay issues (Greene and Herek 1994). However, new British titles are published regularly.

Developing an affirmative therapy approach

Therapy work can be simplified by using an actively anti-oppressive approach. This means identifying the different, though connected, political and social prejudices and discriminations which lesbians have experienced, and avoiding styles of practice which can feel like reinforcement of these oppressions (see also Chapter 2).

The connections are especially well defined in recent books produced by Black lesbians in the UK (Mason-John and Khambatta 1993; Mason-John 1994). Just as racism and sexism have historic connotations for all Black women, for all lesbians sexism and heterosexism are indistinguishable, and ageism can be 'a point of convergence for many other repressive forces' (MacDonald and Rich 1985: 61). The effects of ageism and sexism mean that, when the lesbian image is stereotyped as solely sexual, then 'if old women have no sexuality, it follows that there are no [old] lesbians' (Neild and Pearson 1992: 12). Images of lesbians are excluded even from stereotypes of older women – earth mother, available divorcee, merry widow, mother-in-law, granny, matriarch or 'game old bird'. The few terms which are often euphemisms for older lesbians, such as 'unmarried daughter' imply a caring role and 'maiden aunt' again implies no sexuality.

If heterosexism either pathologizes or renders lesbians invisible (and every gradation between these extremes) ageism does so equally. A 68-year-old lesbian said:

> It feels as if the wheel has turned full circle. I get the same sort of reactions as when I was a young lesbian, and I feel just as vulnerable ... we had no sexuality, no legitimate existence, no support to be ourselves, no needs or rights, and if we came out, no work. I was

discharged from the army as a young lesbian, supposedly for medical reasons.

Older lesbians whose particular needs are overlooked by community organizations may be unable to participate in self-empowering projects or social events, remaining 'forever at the other end of the helping service' (MacDonald and Rich 1985: 65–75). A major change in circumstances can have a profound effect. A 56-year-old lesbian said:

> Being newly disabled following a stroke means, apart from anything else, I'm more dependent on my children. My relationships with lesbian friends have changed dramatically. My daughter is in a way relieved that she can think of me as a granny instead of as a lesbian. I'm respectable, I've even got a sort of status, but it means keeping quiet about the most important part of my life. I'm well looked after, but if I want to go to a gay pub or women's day concert, I have to arrange things with my friends, sneaking around like I did when I was a teenager. My GP has a speech therapist, also a counsellor who is a gay man and is helping me to validate my life. I'm thinking of training to be a telephone bereavement counsellor, which I can do at home.

For women born outside the UK, ageing can increase the awareness of the loss of culture and family roots. An Irish lesbian said: 'I escaped the oppression of Catholicism and settled here, experiencing a lot of prejudice. And ironically so many of my English friends say what a wonderful country Ireland is now for women and lesbians.'

Said an Asian lesbian: 'I worry about getting older, and if we should be so ill that we have to go into supervised care with a lot of white heterosexual men and women, or be separated from each other.' Many Black women have written with great poignancy of how ageing or bereavement intensifies the loss of traditions of respect and care for elders, or of supportive funeral rituals such as the Caribbean nine night wake (Gilroy 1994: 252).

Other Black women have challenged the perception that lesbian sexuality is a white woman's identity, asserting that 'Black lesbians have a long and rich history of being women-identified women in our countries of origin' (Parmar 1989: 221). Equalities trainer Femi Otitojou stated: 'In Nigeria, marrying women is old. It is bush ways' (Mason-John and Khambatta 1993: 19). The experience of racism in majority white lesbian or gay centres 'manifests itself internally and externally as anger, pain, frustration and exhaustion' (Mason-John and Khambatta 1993: 49). Several lesbian or gay organizations, including counselling projects and helplines, are endeavouring to rectify this divisiveness, especially in cities. Enabling clients to recognize the sources of prejudices and their isolating effects is part of effective therapy.

The effects of racism, heterosexism and ageism are of course compounded by other forms of discrimination a lesbian experiences: for instance on the grounds of her ethnicity, class, disability, economic status, appearance, perceived mental health, parental status, faith or political views. In addition, prejudices can be internalized, inherited and socialized, affecting lesbians' relationships with each other, and can have seriously divisive consequences (Mason-John and Khambatta 1993: 45–9). A 56-year-old lesbian who arrived in London in 1960 said: 'I am proud to be an older Black lesbian, but I don't know many others. I wish I knew how we could all contact each other' (Marie 1992: 160).

Therapy issues for older lesbians

Lesbian women share many concerns and experiences with heterosexual women, though there are numerous significant differences. As well as individual issues, there are particular experiences in relationships, work situations, in terms of elders, parenting, adoption or fostering, or feeling acknowledged and valued in the local religious community – often a haven for older people. There are also the double-marginalization issues, such as those experienced by lesbians with disabilities, who again, are often categorized indiscriminately as disabled. Ageism reinforces the traditional perception of women with sensory, physical or learning disabilities as non-sexual and, in lesbian communities, access remains difficult although considerable improvements have been made – including in attitudes – in the past few years.

One such positive story is that of a physically disabled lesbian who said that she felt weird having to explain what her sexual needs were to anyone she wanted to sleep with, until she realized that 'everyone has to explain what their needs are in order to get them met' and that since there is no 'set standard' to lesbian love-making, there is 'a whole world of sexuality and sensuality open to explore' (Phillips and Rakusen 1989: 221).

Challenges presented by social and political changes, the mid-life transition and the menopause have different and additional implications for lesbians.

The challenge of change

Many lesbians' lives (though certainly not all) have been made considerably easier as a result of the changes brought about by the various human rights movements. Others have found developments complex and disorienting. Lesbian politics is constantly changing its focus – for instance, there is a strong anti-therapy movement (Kitzinger and Perkins 1993) and major disagreement about 'appropriate' sexual expression (Jeffreys 1994; McLellan 1995). A 55-year-old lesbian explained:

My identity changed every few years. I was a gay woman, then a lesbian. I was a separatist, then a lesbian–feminist, then a radical dyke. For a while I was a Buddy. The next thing I knew I was back in the women's movement, then there was the backlash. I went into therapy because I felt like just another middle-aged woman going through 'the change' and I didn't want to be there and I wondered where my life had gone.

Language, politics, media, entertainment, sexual health services, fashions, ways of relating and in particular the different approaches to minority lesbian issues, vary considerably from city to city and suburb to suburb. Even a lesbian active and prominent in her own community may develop a new perception of herself on discovering that 'we really do have a different culture from lesbians in their twenties. I always thought the generation gap would never be a problem for me' (Loulan 1991: 10). Many older lesbians prefer to describe a lover or partner as a 'friend' – hence since 1963 the name of the largest national lesbian and gay counselling organization, National Friend – as well as a telling indication of the lesbian relationship ideal of equality. Valuable work can be done by practitioners who are open to sensitive discussion around meanings and implications of self-identifying and politicized terminology.

At the same time as using services, older lesbians may feel grief or resentment about the range available now and denied to them in their younger years. Those who had long term relationships with gay men as friends, co-parents, or companions for family and work events are suffering from the loss of these brothers to AIDS, and feeling left out of gay men's recent focus on legal concerns and their sense of community, or alienated by their sex oriented publications. They may even feel 'survivor guilt', having previously envied gay men's relative freedom and more open and accepted sexuality. Modern feminists now prioritize heterosexual women's concerns.

Mid-life, the menopause, transition and loss

Several factors prompt an individual lesbian to identify new needs, whether or not she perceives these as related to ageing or a 'mid-life' transition, often signalled by the onset of the menopause. Redundancy, the death of a parent or partner, serious and disabling changes in her health or that of a partner or friends, the effects of years of stress from fighting prejudices, or a daughter's first sexual experience, may all be felt as a crisis, even by a usually capable and independent lesbian. This is more likely when events coincide with the profound inner changes of the menopause, as so frequently happens. Tiredness, decreasing well-being, loss of self-confidence and a sense of new vulnerability may lead to the fear of growing old.

While hormone replacement therapy (HRT) has transformed the physical experiences of the menopause, it does not suit all women, requires medical management, and is in some circumstances a health risk. Signs of the menopause appear before decisions about HRT can be taken, as in some cases the symptoms indicate other health problems. Therapists should first avoid labelling all psychological or emotional issues as 'hormone-related', and second avoid interpreting all menopausal mood swings as signs of emotional or psychological disturbances (Young 1995a).

Lesbians share heterosexual women's experiences, for instance, worrying about changes in sexual activities or the risk of hysterectomy or breast cancer, and there are concerns about the ethics of taking HRT because of the implied pathologizing of the menopause and of women's ageing (Fairlie *et al.* 1987: 11–16; Phillips and Rakusen 1989: 453). The popularity of HRT has obscured the fact that the menopause is a natural process, a stage of a woman's sexuality, rather than its termination. Said a 48-year-old lesbian: 'I didn't want to resist or delay the menopause. It felt like a healthy flushing out of old stuff, and a way of finding out why I was so hot and bothered, restless and depressed.'

A sense of separateness from other lesbians can raise memories of coming out and renewed fears of isolation, or of being judged 'sick' or 'crazy'. Alternatively, the menopause can be felt positively like a 'new adolescence' (Barnes and Maple 1992: 74) or yet another 'coming out' (see Chapter 4). However, previously unresolved issues of loss – of community, life structures, security and identity including previous heterosexual identity (Ryan 1983: 199) – can re-emerge.

The loss of a long term partner is traumatic, especially if she was also a business partner or co-parent, and particularly for an isolated lesbian. However, like any bereavement, it may also bring release. These issues can be complicated by the classic menopausal issue of loss – of youth, choices about fertility, experience of sexuality and in some cases, of a 'couple' identity built up through years of struggling for a place and voice. A midmenopausal lesbian explained:

> When my lover died of cancer at 46, I couldn't find any point in being a lesbian. We'd both been so involved in campaigning, years of battling shoulder to shoulder. Friends keep saying, you're a fighter, you'll carry on like you always did, but I haven't the heart. I can't see any results from all that hard work. People can't deal with me being scared and lonely and depressed. They want me to be my old self, but she's not there anymore.

This type of experience can be understood as a lesbian version of the social expectations of all women to 'be there' for other people or for community service, or the importance of being half of a couple, and of being 'not there anymore' as a 'real' woman.

The emotional, psychological and, particularly, sexual implications of the menopause have a different significance for lesbians. A 42-year-old lesbian said:

> My identity as a lesbian was very much about sexuality. Having sex with women was a political statement, it was the one thing we weren't supposed to do. We were strong, we went on marches and demos and discos, we controlled our bodies. The menopause changed all that – I had to have a hysterectomy, and it felt as if I'd lost my sexuality and my power.

Reasons for seeking therapy at mid-life and older are not, of course, solely problem oriented. They can include self-development, focusing on health and future care needs, ending a long term relationship, letting go of old, externally imposed limits on self-expression or finding personal and spiritual purpose and meaning in life (see also Chapter 13). A well-prepared lesbian may feel that ageing brings benefits. Said a 60-year-old:

> I feel more fully a woman and a lesbian without the monthly reminder that I was a mere vulnerable female. I feel I have the right to be an adult, an individual, to be comfortable among and intimate with other lesbians without constant attention to sexual undercurrents. I've accepted an identity for myself as a lesbian that doesn't have to be solely sexual to be valid, and as a woman that doesn't have to be based either on motherhood or being childless. I've accepted what I have instead of worrying about what I don't have.

Conclusions

- The primary purpose of therapy with older lesbians is to support them in countering the effects of a lifetime of oppressions, which should be named as such, and to plan for the future.
- Identity, a major issue in all therapies, is even more crucial for 'lifelong' older lesbians who may never have felt permitted to define themselves.
- An affirmative approach can be underpinned, for instance, by enlisting the client's participation in the choice of methods or techniques and by using her frames of reference and her perspective.
- Identifying a lesbian's previous experiences of dealing with oppressions will enable her to use or adapt these as self-healing tools and to increase self-esteem.
- It is important not to blame emotional and psychological difficulties on the menopause, nor to exclude this as a contributory factor.
- Ageing can be experienced positively when it is not itself problematized, as can the natural menopausal process.

10 | BERNARD RATIGAN

Working with older gay men

This chapter considers some of the themes encountered in psychodynamic counselling and psychotherapy with older gay men. It is a clinical account with no pretensions to be exhaustive. After some introductory material the chapter goes on to consider the need for careful assessment, then looks at questions around ageism, bereavement, internalized homophobia, cultural and ethnic differences and drug use.

Older gay men and therapy

There is as yet very little clinical material published in this area (see Lee 1991; Gutierrez 1992). Most of the clinical work on which the chapter is based is from my work as a psychoanalytic psychotherapist in a specialist public-sector adult psychotherapy service and from a small private practice. The National Health Service unit in which I work receives a considerable number of referrals of gay men (and lesbians). The reasons for this are not altogether clear but may include the willingness of gay, as distinct from heterosexual, men to seek therapeutic help, a possible greater incidence of psychological morbidity (Ross 1988; Catalan 1992) amongst gay men and/or the presence amongst the senior clinical staff of an out gay psychotherapist which perhaps encourages both potential patients to ask for referral and for referrers to refer. This chapter does not consider psychotherapeutic work with lesbians (who are equally well represented in my unit's work) as they are the subject of Chapter 9. As with any writing from a clinical context it is important to stress that my professional experience is with those gay men seeking or being referred for psychotherapeutic help.

The issues being brought by those seeking help *may* be illustrative of the concerns of the wider gay ageing population but extreme caution should be exercised in making generalizations and extrapolations.

The city in which I work, Nottingham, has a very long-established gay culture and scene. I have met many older gay men, patients and non-patients, who have told me of their early lives. Many of the stories are rich in humour, sometimes a little self-parodying and told with considerable dignity. Not all of my witnesses see the growth of a visible, positive gay culture as an unalloyed good thing. I have heard many stories, typically set during World War II or national service, of sexual encounters with so-called heterosexual men who would never define themselves as homosexual or gay (Hall Carpenter Archives 1989). These witnesses sometimes regret much of what they see in the politicization of homosexuality and especially deplore the adoption of the word 'gay'. The politically correct, right-on gay man or 'supportive' heterosexual can be brought up sharply by such attitudes. To explain them away by reductionist accounts, as indicative of internalized homophobia, seems not to take the person seriously and to downgrade the impact of living in a deeply homophobic society such as Britain. One particular issue that sometimes arises in working with older gay men is that of a highly problematic relationship to and with women. Having grown up in social milieu where women were either over-idealized or denigrated, some older gay men have had little exposure to real women, heterosexual or lesbian, as they have lived in mental or physical male ghettos.

In working with gay men of middle and later years it is important to remember that gay cultures have existed for decades, even centuries, and gayness, like sexual intercourse, was decidedly *not* invented in 1963 as the very ungay poet Philip Larkin has it! Although there has been an observable and objective increase in the visibility of white, middle-class, non-disabled gay men since the 1960s, there still remain many other individuals and groups who, like my elderly Nottingham informants, just carry on with their lives. The counsellor or psychotherapist unused to working with gay men would do well to acquaint themselves with the concepts of 'camp' (Sontag 1987) and of 'queer' (Shepherd and Wallis 1989) to better understand their clients.

Therapists of every sexual orientation should keep in mind that throughout most of human history and even now, many men of predominantly homosexual orientation are in heterosexual relationships for whatever reasons and have children (and grandchildren). The desire to have children is, in my view, independent of sexual orientation. What is clear is that we live in a society which accords considerable importance to having children. It is a commonplace that the childless are seen as incomplete people, often needing to justify themselves. In my work I come across examples of gay men of middle and later years who have regrets that they have not fathered children; I also meet many more for whom it is no problem whatsoever. It is unhelpful to have assumptions of what *a* gay man is, or looks like, as far as counselling and psychotherapy are concerned, as the dynamics of non-stereotypical gay men are more likely to be missed. In the 1950s, when West (1955) wrote his ground-breaking book on homosexuality he was able, in a few paragraphs, to draw up a couple of pen portraits of homosexual 'types' which might just have been adequate then but have now been considerably overtaken. No longer is it possible, or wise, to make assumptions about what is *a* homosexual. We now know that there are many 'types' of homosexualities, just as there are 'types' of heterosexualities, and that any sound clinical work needs to recognize this fact and be informed of the range and diversity to be found among gay people (see, for example, Bell and Weinberg 1978).

What is clear is that many outward manifestations of gay male culture appear to overvalue youth and good looks. Of course, this is a superficial, commercially driven imperative but it nevertheless represents a powerful shaper of the internal realities of gay men. It can be seen as but an intensification of the cult of youth and invisibility of the middle aged and especially the old in our society. Put simply, the older you are the less you exist. It is certainly the reported experience of many of the middle aged and older gay men who seek therapy that they often feel alienated from commercial and other gay scenes which overvalue, if not idolize, the young and the beautiful. As Scott Capurro, the American gay comedian, has it, 'Thirty equals eighty in gay years.'

At the level of the individual, these cultural and social attitudes are sometimes translated into an internalized self-alienation which can further serve to isolate the gay man of middle or later years. Research in this field has shown that whilst gay men define for themselves the beginning of middle and old age at roughly the same time as heterosexual men, they see *other* gay men as defining middle and old age beginning some years' earlier (Bennett and Thompson 1991). Clinical practice and personal experience tends to confirm this research finding. One of the tasks of counselling or therapy can be to help the patient see what their assumptive world (Frank 1963) is with regard to age.

Often the ageism so prevalent in the commercial gay world is, perhaps not surprisingly, mirrored and can be found embedded and resonating with patients' internal worlds. It can be very hard to shift and can, in principle, respond much better to group rather than individual intervention (Yalom 1985). My clinical intuition is that gay men do not usually do well in 'mixed' psychotherapy groups (i.e. containing both gays and heterosexuals) except where the group is relatively mature, the therapists exceptionally gay affirmative and sensitive and the gay patient can resist, or be helped to resist, an overly educative role in relation to the other members and the therapists. As with ethnic minority group patients it can be very difficult being put in, or taking on the role of, representative for a whole community, especially saying anything which brings the community into disrepute (but see Helfand 1993). Group analysis remains a problematic area for gay men (Roberts and Pines 1991).

The need for careful assessment

As this chapter is written from a psychodynamic standpoint great emphasis is placed on careful assessment *before* counselling or psychotherapy is recommended or attempted. It is foolishly naïve and cruelly over-optimistic to assume that any kind of psychological intervention can only be benign and always have a good outcome. We live in an age and society which increasingly sees counselling, and to a lesser extent psychotherapy, almost as panaceas for any emotional trauma or distress. I do not share this view and believe it seriously and patronizingly to undervalue human beings' capacity for doing things for themselves and with others, such as friends or relatives, without the benefit of professional intervention. It also gives an unjustifiable amount of power to counselling and psychotherapy.

When working with younger people it may be reasonable to assume a degree of therapeutic optimism, but once we start working with people who have reached chronological, if not developmental, maturity it is much harder to change. Major life events and processes such as the loss of one, or even worse both, parents in childhood, separation from parents, histories of abuse, drug misuse or deliberate self-harm, profound social isolation, long histories of mental illness and previous unsuccessful attempts at counselling or psychotherapy should all signal caution to a counsellor or psychotherapist considering taking someone on. Particular care needs to be exercised when prospective clients have narcissistic or borderline personality disorders as they will often need intensive help and those treating them may well need specialist supervision (Silverstein 1988). In considering taking on the older gay man for counselling or therapy, it is important to make as thorough an assessment as is possible and be modest in one's therapeutic goals. The impact of having lived an emotionally and socially impaired life in a homophobic culture makes major change unlikely. Some change is often possible but the old medical dictum of 'at least do no harm' should guide the work.

Case examples

There follows a number of fictional short case examples which illustrate the range of counselling and psychotherapeutic interventions with older gay men.

Case example 1: internalized ageism

Jack, a gay man in his late 40s, in therapy because of an unusual number of significant losses in his life, told his therapist he was unhappy at what others thought about his having a partner much younger than himself as well as several other very close friends and lovers in their 20s and 30s.

The therapist acknowledged his anxieties as well as helping understand the roots of this and also pointed out he had many friends in their 50s, 60s, 70s and even 80s. This helped the client to begin to see his internalized ageism and the fact that he had a very wide age-range of friends. He was also able to begin to explore at a deeper level the links between his concern about ageing, his own mortality, his partner's fears about what would happen after his (the patient's) death and other existential and eschatological themes. It is rare for gay patients to present with *ageing*, as such, as a problem when coming forward for counselling or psychotherapy. It is much more likely to emerge as work unfolds and can provide a fruitful focus of work. Psychodynamic and other forms of counselling and psychotherapy have within their repertoires of discourse understandings surrounding death and the search for meaning which can help gay men (Yalom 1980; Spinelli 1989).

Concerns surrounding death and meaning have become much sharper and more relevant since the onset of HIV in the 1980s. There can be few gay men left now in Britain whose lives have not been affected by HIV. Indeed, there are gay men coming forward for counselling or therapy who could be described as suffering from survivor guilt and other forms of post-traumatic stress disorder because they have lost so many of their partners and friends. Many will have heard the words of the Psalmist, 'Media vita ... In the midst of life we are in death' spoken at the funeral services of lovers and friends and, even though they may not be Jews or Christians, will know the truth of it. Some will be thinking that they too face an early death. Others will perhaps smile at the thought that some gay men are actually worried about getting old and wish they could be so fortunate.

Case example 2: bereavement

Tom, a 49-year-old gay man, was referred for therapy by his genitourinary health adviser after losing his partner of over 20 year's standing. Although they had never lived together they had seen each other, in Tom's words, as 'an item', and had been so seen by their friendship network. Tom's partner had died from an HIV related illness and had been devotedly looked after by Tom until his death about two months before the referral. After his partner's funeral, which had been attended by many people from their friendship network, the neighbourhood and the wider gay community, Tom was unable to readjust to normal life. He had lost other significant people in his life, including his own parents and other friends from HIV and other illnesses, and he had an expectation that he should soon be getting back to normal. Sleeplessness, frequent tears and what he called an 'aching emptiness' pervaded his life. He went to his sympathetic GP and was given a 'sick note' and advised to look for a new partner. When the GU health adviser gave him a routine phone call to check how he was, Tom poured out his pain to her and she arranged to see him for supportive counselling. The health adviser discussed his difficulties in supervision and a decision was made to seek specialist help for him from a psychotherapist.

After assessment by the psychotherapist, weekly sessions commenced which Tom used to explore more deeply the range of feelings of loss that had been released by his partner's death. Most notable was his rage at his partner for getting infected with HIV in the first place. Whilst the partner was alive, they had never really aired the whole subject of the infection because Tom was, he said, frightened about looking at the truth. The partner's death also evoked considerable feelings about both Tom's parents' deaths and about his own life. As the therapy unfolded he was able to get in touch with long-buried feelings of rage and depression going back to his childhood and his first attempts at coming out. He became actively suicidal for a period in the therapy and was started on concurrent anti-depressant medication. Over a period of months he gradually was able to work through the bereavement and after a year of sessions he was able to move toward termination, apparently having gained new strengths and insights into himself and his loss (Raphael 1984; Lendrum and Syme 1994).

Case example 3: I'm not gay, I'm queer

Quentin, a man of 72 years, asked for counselling after getting upset when an ex-parish priest of his received newspaper publicity over an allegation of possessing paedophile pornography. He spoke of his shock at what he had experienced as a betrayal of trust by the priest. He explained to the counsellor that he had no truck with such words as gay and preferred to think, but never to speak, of himself as queer. In this he predated by many decades the recent rehabilitation of the word, except he used it in a highly pejorative sense. His life as a single man who lived with his parents until they died in his 50s and 60s was one of quiet desperation. He told the counsellor he had never, consciously, known any other gay man or lesbian. He had always owed strong and partisan allegiance to the high church wing of the Church of England.

Working with older gay men 165

In counselling, Quentin began to find a voice for his distress and to express his envious rage that so much of his life had, in his words, been wasted. He spoke to the counsellor about his one experience of freedom during World War II when he felt free to be sexual. Since then he had eschewed any sexual contact, wanting to believe that if he did he would ensure his place in heaven. Now he was less sure. The publicity given to his priest had shaken the very roots of his existence. Perhaps the most significant area of work for Quentin was his starting to unravel his relationship with his mother, whom he had previously always idolized. In counselling, he came to see a less over-idealized aspect of his mother. What made it particularly hard for the counsellor was coping with Quentin's bitterness and the withering attacks he constantly made on the values of the counsellor. The counsellor was able, for the most part, to contain his own retaliatory hatred in the counter-transference in the belief that this was what usually happened in Quentin's abortive relationships, allowing him to carry on with his bitter, feeling-sorry-for-himself life. Over time, Quentin became a little less bitter with the counsellor and allowed more of his sadness to emerge. He died from a massive heart attack after about a year's work and the counsellor joined the very small congregation at his funeral.

Case example 4: the spy who came out of the closet

Errol, a 48-year-old man of African-Caribbean background, was referred for psychotherapy by his GP from whom he had sought help with symptoms of depression. On assessment he painfully told the psychotherapist of his recently growing realization that he was gay, finding it hard to put his thoughts and feelings into words. He had found himself increasingly drawn to visit a porno cinema in another town and having anonymous sex with the other male patrons.

Making a therapeutic relationship with Errol was a very difficult task. He had hidden his homosexuality from himself and from the world since before puberty and had 'passed' as a heterosexual to the extent of fathering three children. He felt very threatened because, as he admitted once therapy commenced, for many years he had really believed that there were no black gay men and had taken a leading role in his workplace in castigating his white colleagues who showed any sign of effeminacy or weakness. In the safety of the therapeutic relationship he was able to see how he had organized most of his life as an elaborate charade, saying that he felt like a spy in an enemy country.

Amongst his many worries was the impact of his homosexuality becoming known amongst his family and community. He feared total rejection and losing contact with his children and his family network. When he found the courage to go to a gay club in a city many miles away he was shaken when he bumped into a distant cousin. What seemed to precipitate his depressive symptoms was the coming out of a well-known black sportsman whom Errol had long admired and the happenstance meeting with his distant gay cousin.

The question of the different racial identities of the patient and the psychotherapist was ever present in the mind of the psychotherapist who took every opportunity to raise it. Errol's view was that he did not want to see a black clinician, gay or heterosexual, nor was he prepared to have any truck with voluntary community groups which he castigated because he perceived them as being run by white middle-class people. After a year of therapy, free of symptoms, he announced he had met a gay white man and wanted to stop seeing the psychotherapist, which he did. At the six month follow-up, Errol reported that he was still in a relationship with his new friend and they had decided to go into business, but not live, together. He remained psychiatrically asymptomatic and was considering offering himself to train as a buddy in an HIV voluntary organization. His earlier writing-off of gay groups as irredeemably bourgeois and white seemed to have been somewhat altered by first-hand experience.

Thinking about Errol, a number of points come to mind. Bion (1965), the Kleinian psychoanalyst, wrote of the need to attempt to enter every session without memory, desire or will. With Errol, the psychotherapist was often conscious of having projects for him: get him to talk about the ethnic differences between them, to try to get Errol linked up with other black gay men, etc. What seems of greatest interest is Errol's developed capacity for not knowing. He was able to turn a blind eye to his homosexuality over many years and perhaps used his virulent attacks on his white peers as a way of shoring up his inner confusion and doubt. Once he was confronted by a high profile black out gay man, in the shape of his sporting hero, and spotting his cousin whom he assumed to be gay because he saw him in a gay club, the carapace protecting his real sexual orientation began to crack and he developed depressive symptoms which his GP was able to read correctly and make an appropriate referral. Once again, the therapeutic task had to be sensitive to the decades of repression which this man had experienced and the racial and cultural realities of his world and not push him too much so as to avoid the risk of flight or decompensation into a much more serious mental illness. The question of his relationships with the mother of his children and with his children remained a continuing source of considerable tension but one with which he felt better able to cope.

Case example 5: alcohol as antidepressive
Alcohol has traditionally played quite a prominent role in gay culture both on the commercial scene and in domestic settings. Chapter 11 discusses issues arising from alcohol, and other substance use, in detail.

Charles, a 60-year-old gay man, was referred by his GP for a psychotherapy consultation to determine if anything could be done to help him reduce his drinking as it was seriously threatening to shorten his life. When Charles saw the psychotherapist for assessment he asked if his partner Barry, who was aged 55, could also be involved in the treatment. He argued that they were a couple and had been so for over 20 years, and should be seen together.

There are numerous models of couple therapy and the one adopted in this instance was informed by psychodynamic theory and practice. From a gay affirmative, systemic perspective, Carl (1990) is an invaluable starting point whilst Ruszczynski (1993) provides a psychoanalytic account out of the experience of the Institute of Marital Studies at the Tavistock Clinic in London. Both men were eventually seen individually by different psychotherapists and then the couple and the two psychotherapists started a series of joint meetings. Amongst the themes that found voice with Charles and Barry were: the reason why Charles drank so much, his inability to speak of his great hurt at being left for weeks at a time whilst Barry was away working in the oil exploration industry and Barry's guilt at the sexual encounters he had whilst away. After a relationship lasting for more than 20 years the two said they found the half dozen joint psychotherapy sessions very frightening but important in attempting to bring some life back into their relationship because it gave them some neutral space in which to talk and think together. After the couple work ended, Charles decided to seek individual psychotherapy to work on his own feelings about the relationship and to help him keep his alcohol consumption at a low to moderate level.

Conclusions

This short chapter has illustrated some of the range of clinical work undertaken with gay men in middle and later life. It takes for granted that gay affirmative psychotherapy and counselling are available increasingly (in major cities) in Britain. There is still considerable work to be done to train mental health professionals as well as community and voluntary agencies in the special features of working with gay and lesbian patient populations. The counselling world seems to consider that it has little or no problem with homosexuality but, as we have seen in Part I of this book, this is probably a self-deluding fiction in such a homophobic culture as Britain. Recent papers in the psychotherapy and psychoanalytic journals indicate that homosexuality remains particularly problematic for the London-based psychoanalytic establishment which continues to see it as inherently pathological; see Hildebrand (1992), Limentani (1994) and Burgner (1994) for examples of the way homosexuality is viewed by some psychoanalytic writers. In contrast there have been some outstanding lesbian affirmative critiques such as O'Connor and Ryan (1993). Following the success of the feminist critique of Freud and his followers, Friedman (1988), Lewes (1988), Isay (1989), Beard and Glickauf-Hughes (1994) and Stubrin (1994) all provide reworkings of the highly negative and dangerous psychoanalytic accounts of male homosexuality in attempts to make it more useful to gay men.

Among the particular areas needing research in therapeutic work with older gay men are the impact of multiple losses being sustained in the wake of the HIV epidemic, appropriate interventions to help combat substance abuse, especially alcohol, and the establishment of couple counselling and therapy facilities. There is much work to be done.

My final thoughts are about the role of friendship in gay men's lives. It is my contention that what best makes for mental health in gay men is to be out of the closet and have a wide circle of good friends to love and be nourished by. Gay people seem to have more opportunities than heterosexuals to have quality friendships with both other gay people and heterosexuals. This may be because we are freed from some of the constraints of heterosexism and have learned that trying to curry favour with an oppressive, macho, homophobic culture by remaining in the closet does not make for happiness, only a pseudo-respectability. By coming out we are challenged to make our own partnerships and friendships freed from many of the conventions of those around us. It is a challenge which needs courage to take up and maintain. Counselling and psychotherapy have parts to play in helping some gay men to make and sustain friendships and relationships and improve the quality of the middle and later years.

- Older clients, having adopted different strategies for living in a homophobic society, sometimes regret the increased visibility, politicization and overtness of contemporary 'gay' cultures.
- Many older gay men have lived in mental or physical male ghettos.
- Internalized self-alienation, exacerbated by cultural or internalized ageism, can further isolate gay men of middle and later years.
- There can be problems for gay men in mixed therapy groups.
- Therapists need to make thorough assessments before working with older men, not all of whom can benefit, and to keep therapeutic goals modest.
- HIV has contributed powerfully to gay men's concerns with death and meaning, few having been unaffected in some way and many suffering forms of post-traumatic stress disorder.
- Decades of repression lead sometimes to highly developed capacities for not knowing; it is important to respect such defences and sensitively avoid pushing clients into flight responses or decompensation and, thereby, more serious mental illness.

- Psychoanalysis continues to pathologize homosexuality while more recent critiques have contributed positively to reworking homophobic models. Much work remains to be done in research and clinical practice.

Acknowledgements

I would like to thank my partner Paul Wishart, patients, colleagues, friends and especially Dr Peter Wilson for help with this chapter. It could not have been written without them.

11 | GRAZ KOWSZUN AND MAEVE MALLEY

Alcohol and substance misuse

First, the disclaimers: to have a chapter about issues of lesbian and gay men's substance use might seem to imply that we form a homogenous group, which of course we do not. We may define ourselves much more in terms of our gender, race, class, age, nationality or disability than our sexuality. We may see our substance use as entirely unconnected to our background, or see it as familially, culturally or occupationally based, connected or unconnected to our sexuality, as positive or negative.

'Substance use' in this context covers the use of a whole spectrum of mood altering drugs (prescribed or unprescribed) including all types of alcohol. Strictly speaking, this would include tobacco, tea and coffee, but we will be focusing on drugs more obviously perceived as intoxicants.

We also need to define just who we are talking about; by 'lesbians' and 'gay men' we will take to mean those who so define themselves or whose primary sexual orientation is towards their own gender. Bisexuals may, according to their own definitions, identify more or less with some of the specifics applicable to lesbians and gay men. Our experience is primarily in working with lesbians, gay men and heterosexuals, rather than with people who self-define as bisexual, so there may be very different conditions applying to bisexuals that we are not qualified to discuss. Consequently, we don't propose to append, 'and bisexuals' every time we are talking about lesbians and gay men – they deserve a discrete piece of work – but we shall be very happy if any of this seems relevant to bisexuals.

Defining the issue

Drinking and drug use are widespread in white western cultures and not noticeably absent from any culture. The mood-changing substances used vary, but most fall within the categories of depressants, narcotic analgesics, stimulants or hallucinogens. Most drugs can be used therapeutically and recreationally, some are legal and ubiquitous, some are illegal and more or less easy to acquire. Alcohol is the drug most obviously interwoven into the fabric of white western industrialized culture and causes the greatest damage, in terms of numbers affected. It is the drug used by most people and the degree of social acceptability given to it tends to make us underrate what a powerful drug it is, with a very high capacity to create physical dependence. In considering the numbers of people affected by substance abuse we must include not only the drinker or drug user, but also their past and present lovers, family, friends and colleagues.

Society protects itself from awareness of its own ambivalence regarding substance use by categorizing people who experience problems with their use as in some way 'deviant' or 'different'; terms such as 'alcoholic' or 'junkie' separate such people out from the population in general. *Everyone* has the potential to use mood-changing substances and the potential to run into difficulties with that use. Many people have problems with their use at some times in their life and no problems at all at other times.

It is also worth saying here that many of us who use, or have used, alcohol or drugs extensively have done so because it can be fun to do so. Substance use is not just about fulfilling unmet needs, blanking out unhappiness or compensating for the inadequacy of relationships. It can, of course, be about these negative things and, unfortunately, the heavier the use, the more the user will tend to experience negative effects, and therefore use more to compensate for them and so on. There are, however, no real givens about what creates problematic use; society has regarded substance use in various ways at various times. It is worth surveying these models briefly, if only to realize that they are 'models' and not truths and because, as therapists, we have all internalized these models to some degree.

Models of use

In the last three centuries in Western Europe and North America, the general societal stance towards drinkers and drug users has shifted perceptibly from a moral to a medical model. There seems to be a current (1996) shift to a more fundamentalist Christian stance on alcohol and drug use, exemplified by the 'Twelve-Step' philosophy so popular in the United States (i.e. Alcoholics Anonymous, Narcotics Anonymous). Interesting parallels can be seen between models of drink and drug use and models which seek to 'explain' homosexuality. They have, generally, both moved from the eighteenth- and early nineteenth-century mode of regarding drinkers/users and lesbians/gay men as imbued with a moral weakness or vice, to seeing us as less 'bad' than 'mad' or 'sad'. There are stalwart defenders of the 'bad' theory in outposts of bigotry (as discussed in Part I) but, with the rise of the medico-scientific establishment in the nineteenth and twentieth centuries, the perception of both groups as 'ill' (and therefore to be pitied as well as abused) has gained acceptability. Disease, allergy, early trauma, physiological structure, genetic predisposition, all have been cited as 'causal'. It is difficult to know if this has had many positive effects in terms of how people are treated but, despite sterling efforts and great financial investment, no such 'causal' factors have been reputably proven in the fields of either drink and drug use or sexuality.

In the 1960s a new formulation of drug and alcohol use began to be discussed by psychologists, workers and theorists based on the ideas of social learning theorists (genesis discussed in Heather and Robertson 1989). Put simply, these describe problematic drug use as the result of learned patterns, which can, consequently, be 'unlearned'. This model undermines the notion of a 'disease' in which abstinence is the only 'cure'. It introduces a much less absolutist attitude into treatment methodologies; this may be why it has yet to be absorbed into the mainstream thinking on substance use.

Choice of theory or model is just that – a choice – substantiated by one's own experience. Accuracy or 'truth' is in the eye of the beholder. If a 'problem' drinker or drug user believes that their substance use is genetically determined, or a disease, and that abstinence is the only option, they may find it constructive to use Alcoholics Anonymous or Narcotics Anonymous support groups, which also hold to a 'disease model'. Conversely, if they feel that this view is too simplistic and want to alter, rather than necessarily cease, their use, they can find many agencies who can provide group or individual support or counselling based on this approach. Provided that our formulations work for us – i.e. they give us a reasonable sense of self-efficacy and do not imbue us with feelings of guilt or self-hatred – it is probably irrelevant what we believe.

What is important, is that lesbians and gay men who have, or have had, any problems associated with drink or drug use, and those who are working in a helping role with them and their significant others, should be aware that there is no one 'true way' of dealing with those problems and it should never be a condition of help that any belief has to be accepted or rejected.

Is substance use a particular issue for lesbians and gay men?

There are several reasons for considering that substance use is an issue for lesbians and gay men. First, there seems to be a strong possibility that lesbians and gay men are overrepresented in the population reporting problems with alcohol and drug use (see Fifield 1975; Lohrenz *et al.* 1978; Stall and Wiley 1988; McKirnan and Peterson 1989). There are various theories of why this may be so, which we will be reviewing. Second, lesbians and gay men need to take on more than average responsibility for our own well-being and for getting appropriate and useful assistance in promoting that well-being.

In other words, lesbians and gay men are not, and have never been, well-served by physical and mental health professionals and institutions. So, in studies, more lesbians and gay men report more problems with their substance use. Yet anecdotal evidence from British alcohol services (most services do not monitor the sexuality of their clients) and American commentators (Straub in Burtle 1979; Sandmaier 1980) suggests that proportionally fewer lesbians and gay men than the general population use the services available. This may also indicate that lesbians and gay men who do use the services do not identify their sexuality.

This general wariness of services (or of being 'out' when using services) probably stems from a perception of the possibility of encountering homophobic, or otherwise unhelpful, attitudes. It can be argued that the 'helping' professions are slightly less homophobic than some other areas of work, but they have their fair share and, as discussed in earlier chapters, the medical and psychiatric establishments generally have nurtured some unthinking attitudes and abusive practices. Later we will discuss ways to avoid perpetuating bigoted attitudes in work with substance users who want help.

In looking at the incidence of lesbians and gay men who may have problems associated with substance use, research is sketchy and potentially misleading. A certain amount of research has been done on drinking and drug use among lesbians and gay men, though the situation has not changed radically since Peter Nardi (1982: 9) stated,

> The *Journal of Studies on Alcohol* is one of the most important publications in the alcohol field... From 1951 through 1980, however, there were only 42 references under the heading of homosexuality.

A small number of studies are consistently cited in the literature; these are in 1970 and 1973 by Saghir and Robins; 1975 by Fifield; 1978 by Lohrenz *et al.*; 1978 by Diamond and Wilsnack; 1988 by Stall and Wiley; and 1988 and 1989 by McKirnan and Peterson. There will, of course, have been studies done since then but certainly these are the ones quoted and requoted in the literature. It is enormously important that these studies have been done – anything that adds to the knowledge base and is not biased by homophobia or false assumptions needs to be cherished – but the conclusions are limited and very often the limitations are not pointed out.

Kristine Falco (1991: 149) is a notable exception when she says, 'Most studies lack control groups, lack a representation of a cross-section of gays and lesbians and rely upon self-report.' These limitations affect the accuracy of the data gathered, particularly since the majority of the studies focused on white, middle-class, mid-30s, North American gay men – not an entirely representative group!

Nevertheless, while the results from these studies must be regarded with caution, and at least one more recent, though small-scale, study would seem to contradict conclusions about rates of lesbian drinking from earlier studies (Bloomfield 1993), the findings are disturbing. Compared to a 1982 study of the US general population where 8 per cent of women and 16 per cent of men reported having had problems with alcohol (Clark and Midanik 1982), findings from these studies of lesbians varied from figures of 23 per cent to 35 per cent having, or having had, problems with alcohol use. Among gay men, the percentage varied in a range from 19 per cent to 30 per cent reporting such problems.

Within the lesbian and gay population there is, as compared with the heterosexual population, considerable divergence with regard to how gender and age affect drinking practices. McKirnan and Peterson (1989: 549) say, in referring to their study of 3400 lesbians and gay men (22 per cent women, 78 per cent men), as compared to a general population sample,

> Younger males from the two samples showed very similar problem rates. However, the percentage of general population males showing problems substantially decreased in the older age groups, as is commonly found. In contrast, homosexual males showed far less decrease in problem rates over age. Homosexual women reported more symptoms in all age groups and as with males, showed far less decrease across age than the general population.

Clearly then, while heterosexual men drink less as they grow older, the same does not apply to gay men or to lesbians.

Not surprisingly then, with regard to drinking, lesbians interpret their gender roles differently than heterosexual women and are subject to different constraints. Older lesbians and gay men seem to feel that when it comes to alcohol and drug use, they can respond differently to growing older than do heterosexuals, that they don't have to take on certain roles or ways of behaving. Heterosexual drinking patterns may vary more widely than is generally assumed, however, as demonstrated by Cochrane's (1989) study, which indicates that older (over 40) Asian men in Britain consume more alcohol than Asian men under 40, which is directly opposed to the trend in the white population (Cochrane 1989).

If we accept that lesbians and gay men report higher rates of drinking and higher rates of problems connected with drinking than in the general population, we need to look first at whether that correlates with studies on other drug use among lesbians and gay men and second, at why this might be so. On the first point, Stall and Wiley say,

> Among the homosexual and heterosexual samples as a whole, gay men are significantly more likely to use marijuana, poppers, MDA, psychedelics, barbiturates, ethyl chloride and amphetamines.
> ... based on the data from this study, it is probably reasonable to include urban gay men among the list of social groups characterized by exceptionally heavy rates of drug use, with the understanding that the question of whether gay men are characterized by high prevalence rates for problematic substance use remains open.
> (Stall and Wiley 1988: 68, 71)

The 1989 McKirnan and Peterson study tended to support these findings in a mixed gender sample. They say,

> Substantially higher proportions of the homosexual sample used alcohol, marijuana and cocaine than was the case in the general population. Contrary to other reports, this was not accompanied by higher rates of heavy use, though homosexuals did show higher rates of alcohol problems. In the general population, women consume less drugs and alcohol than do men and substance use substantially declines with age. Neither of these patterns were found for the homosexual sample, thus creating higher rates of substance abuse. This may reflect differences between homosexuals and the general population in their adherence to sex-role stereotypes and age-related social changes as well as culturally specific stressors and vulnerability to substance use.
> (McKirnan and Peterson 1989: 545)

These findings apply to North American settings and are difficult to compare to research in other countries, since so little other work has been done, but anecdotal evidence in England seems to support the American findings on alcohol and drug use. We need many more well-conducted research studies before we can draw any truly reliable conclusions, but generally, it does seem that lesbians and gay men drink more and experience more problems with their alcohol use than the heterosexual population. We also seem to use drugs more widely and over a longer period of years than the heterosexual population.

Various causes have been cited to explain these higher rates of use. There are, of course, classic psychoanalytic and medical explanations, which tend to be highly damning – oral fixations, lack of emotional development and general perversity. Ignoring these as serious contenders, theories tend to fall within the frameworks of sociocultural and learning theory. These regard the bar-oriented gay social settings as reinforcing to high levels of alcohol and drug use. In terms of access to alcohol and drug use, gay men tend to have higher disposable incomes than the general population, though this is not the case with lesbians, who may be more liable to be in full time, paid work than heterosexual women, and still end up at the bottom of the economic ladder (Bloomfield 1993).

Other causal factors cited include the experience of external and internalized homophobia and heterosexism, the related stress and the need to feel confident and assertive in an unwelcoming society. Since lesbians and gay men need to make conscious choices and efforts to meet lovers and form peer groups, this requires that we take the risk of going to a gay venue or otherwise letting ourselves be identified as lesbian or gay. We often need to combine this with great circumspection in discussing our personal lives with friends, colleagues and families. This possible isolation and anticipation of attack or rejection does not combine easily with the amount of self-esteem needed to deal with the hurdles presented in meeting a supportive group of peers or lovers. Many lesbians and gay men will have been drinking or drug-using on the first occasion that we have sex with a person of the same gender. While this can feel helpful in terms of the (socially constructed, rather than actually physiological) disinhibiting effects, it can also lead to the sense of this being something that we only do when we're drunk or stoned – therefore the drug use can remain in some way separate from our sense of ourselves as a whole. This combination is also a highly unhelpful factor in terms of keeping an awareness of safer sex on the agenda. There is evidence from studies, such as the long term research Project Sigma, investigating gay male sexual behaviour patterns, that alcohol and drugs used to alter moods also alter sexual practices with a greater emphasis on those which are less safe.

There is the possibility that the pattern of independent thought needed to entertain the idea of being lesbian or gay tends to persist in other aspects of our lives – in other words, that we do not rely on received wisdom or social constraints and respond more easily to notions of personal, rather than social, authority. This can make us creative, innovative and risk taking in positive ways, but lays us open to vulnerabilities associated with risky behaviour and the possible desire for immediate gratification.

In the short term, drink and drug use can boost our sense of self-efficacy, our confidence, our feeling of personal power – all things that feel particularly necessary in a homophobic and misogynist world which can continually batter our self-esteem. Heavy or very regular use will, in the long term, erode our sense of self. The rejection of socially ascribed age roles, and of gender socialization, may tend to work against us if it means that we use more alcohol and drugs over a longer period of time and are reluctant to seek help.

The general population will do the majority of its alcohol and drug-taking in adolescence and early adulthood, when the likelihood of some types of physical and social damage is cushioned by youth and our culture's expectations of young people. A high proportion of people who have been heavy drinkers or drug users will reduce use in their 30s and early 40s. Since it seems that lesbians and gay men tend to retain higher consumption patterns for longer, older gay men and lesbians of all ages will be more prone to the associated physical, social and occupational problems. Lesbians may well be vulnerable since women have much higher rates of substance-related liver damage and higher alcohol-related morbidity rates than men (Chou 1994).

Anybody anywhere can experience problems of various kinds connected to their own, or another's, substance use, which can damage self-esteem and create guilt and self-hatred very quickly. Consequently, it is crucial that lesbians and gay men should have access to knowledge, information, advice and therapeutic help in whatever form is best and that we feel able to use the appropriate services.

Clinical implications

In the second part of this chapter, we examine practical implications of working with clients' issues relating to substance use, an enormously diverse area both in terms of the client group and the readership of this book.

The client group is diverse in terms of age, race, culture, and lifestyle, the difficulties clients face, the mood altering drugs involved and the individual's involvement in counselling or psychotherapy, among other factors. There will be clients who are aware of a need to explore and change their relationship to intoxicating substances. Others will have pressing needs in this area but will not have identified them and some of these clients may be in counselling or psychotherapy working on other issues. In many cases the worst consequences of the pattern of substance use may be cushioned by others, who may feel powerless to effect any change or be colluding with the problem for conscious or unconscious reasons of their own. These 'significant others' may also be in counselling in their own right. A further group of clients may be using substances in a way which enhances their lives, causing few difficulties other than, for example, through the chemical's illegality or as a result of the disapproval of an actual or internal 'critical parent'. Clients, like most people in every society who use mood altering chemicals, will vary in their preferences. However, there will be differences between the nature of the substance used, its perceived benefits and costs, the nature and urgency of reducing any harm incurred, the support available to the client, the significance of the substance issue in the overall context of the client's current life and the relationship, if any, of all of these factors to the client's sexuality and psychological health.

There is likely to be a similar diversity in the competencies and learning needs of the probable readership of this chapter. In order to work effectively with this client group, the therapist needs commitment, knowledge, certain skills and attitudes and a gay affirmative approach.

Commitment

Above all, the counsellor must develop the will to overcome blocks to good and ethical practice in this area and to meet the cost of that commitment, in terms of energy, time and tangible resources. These blocks will vary widely from therapist to therapist. For example, a therapist who believes it is normal for people, especially men, to drink daily and get drunk occasionally, but views illegal drug-taking as always problematic, is likely to have difficulties developing the necessary depth of understanding or acceptance of a lesbian client who smokes marijuana most weekends, but eschews alcohol and expresses concern about one partner's use of cocaine and another's occasional pub crawls. Alternately, a person-centred or psychodynamic counsellor, who has had a difficult relationship in the past with a client whose attendance was erratic and who used poppers, may overcompensate for their own reactions and use their theoretical approaches as justification for their unwillingness to initiate exploration of substance-related issues with a client who sometimes looks unfocused and possibly stoned. Overcoming such blocks is likely to involve self-challenge and change with all its implications for the individual practitioner, and it may involve challenging the policies and practices of institutions in which the therapist works or from which they get support.

Knowledge

An adequate knowledge base may take some time to acquire, and access to an experienced practitioner as well as appropriate training and material is strongly recommended. The therapist needs to know about the common mood altering drugs used in this society. This knowledge should cover their form, availability, method of use and cost. It is also important to have a sense of likely attitudes to the substance within both the mainstream culture and the social milieu of the client. What are the substances' desired effects, possible consequences of intoxication and likely effects of long term or heavy use on health, the psyche, relationships and life in general? Is it a substance which creates physical dependency and if so, how is its degree and severity assessed? What are the withdrawal symptoms and what treatment is available to overcome physical dependency? What are the common strategies and approaches used to tackle problems created by that particular substance and their likely efficacy and appropriateness for different client groups? What other resources are available locally in terms of referring on or working alongside? Where can sound, helpful and up to date information be found for both the client and counsellor? Who can provide consultancy and emotional support for the therapist? To whom else might the client be able to turn for assistance, either formally or informally? If there are additional support networks for the client, what is the theory and practice of these networks – are they gay affirmative? – and what are the likely benefits and limitations for different client groups? The bibliography and resources lists at the end of this book include helpful organizations and introductory books we would recommend to practitioners who want to take a first step to increase their knowledge base.

Skills

The counsellor needs specific skills to assess the impact of the substance use, where the client is in the process of overcoming the issue, and how to work effectively with the client to achieve their desired outcome. These skills, described in more detail in the introductory texts listed in Appendix 3, include specific assessment, monitoring and evaluating skills, as well as ways and means to explore personal meanings of particular patterns of use. There are the skills of motivational interviewing, relapse prevention, of designing and effectively using diaries, decision making charts and cue and consequence analyses. There are also skills in developing client ownership of goals, non-judgemental exploration, awareness and use of countertransference and many others.

Theory of counselling and psychotherapy

The practitioner's core theoretical model may need to be integrated with an approach that allows for specific work with the substance use on the levels of cognition and behaviour as well as exploration of its meaning, consequences and underlying causes. Sometimes a client will make the necessary behavioural changes of their own accord as a result of the work they do at other levels; however this should not be assumed. A gay affirmative value-base is also essential in order not to add to the difficulties of those struggling with issues arising from sexual orientation and substance use on top of other life stresses.

Attitudes

This includes awareness of both the counsellor's own attitudes, assumptions and issues relating to sexual orientation and substance use and also of what attitudes are culturally prevalent, and hence what the client may be expecting or fearing.

Principles of good practice

Clearly, readers will have different degrees of competence with regard to the previous five areas and widely different learning needs. Space does not permit us to address any of these in depth so we shall limit ourselves to suggesting some general principles and refer those interested to other sources for further information. These principles, which are by no means exhaustive, can be considered under six headings, which we shall now address in turn.

The importance of exploring the client's relation to substance use

Whatever the context in which you work, be aware that the client's relation to substance use may be an issue. Develop appropriate ways to assess this, both initially with the client and as their story unfolds. Use supervision to explore possible issues and identify sensitive means of checking these out with the client.

Possible questions to consider under this heading are as follows:

- What are the possible substance-related issues and for whom are they issues (for example, for the client, significant others in the client's life, the counsellor)?
- Whose use of substances may be problematic for the client? Could it be the client, the current partner, colleagues or friends, family or significant people in the client's past, or a combination?
- Given the client's life experience, what conclusions may they have drawn concerning the benefits and costs of using particular substances?
- In both the short and longer term, what does the client perceive as the advantages and disadvantages of addressing each of their substance-related issues?
- What might it take to resolve each issue, partially and fully?
- What are the consequences of *not* addressing these issues for the client and also for the counselling relationship?
- How might you prioritize with the client the issues to address?
- What resources and support do you need to work effectively with your client on these issues?

Case example 1
This example illustrates some of the ways that the thread of substance use may weave through a client's life history. Imagine yourself to be Rupert's

Alcohol and substance misuse

counsellor and consider what the issues may be and how you might approach them?

> Rupert has been seeing a counsellor for six months to deal with the impact of childhood abuse. His father was a heavy drinker, an angry and violent man. His mother was depressed and dependent on tranquillizers. Rupert's half-brother, eight years older than him and currently described by Rupert as a 'speed freak', paid him more attention than either parent; however, that attention included sexual abuse. Rupert has been regularly involved in relationships with men who drink heavily, and has a firm belief that his love will heal them. His current partner is in counselling and making good progress in substantially controlling his drinking. However, their relationship is becoming so fraught that Rupert feels lost, confused and very anxious. This is affecting his work where he is in conflict with his line manager, and the only way Rupert finds he can relax is by going out to visit friends of his with whom he smokes cannabis.

As you examined this vignette in terms of the questions suggested earlier, there are many possible substance issues you may have identified. The alcohol use of his father, previous partners and current partner is problematic for Rupert. His current partner is clearly addressing this and that may be creating difficulties for Rupert. Rupert has made a point of mentioning his half-brother's use of stimulants (with the attendant possible contrast to the depressive effect of alcohol or his mother's tranquillizers), and Rupert's own use of cannabis and choice of a marijuana-smoking peer group could also be explored. Rupert's behaviour is certainly suggesting ambivalence. Is he recreating the environment in which he grew up, where contact with natural moods was perhaps rare and even more dangerous (as in his half-brother's sexual abuse) than being among the intoxicated? Perhaps he could fear, or feel unable to face, change or anxiety without recourse to mood altering substances? Certainly, further exploration of the conclusions the child Rupert may have drawn about both the dangers of intimacy and the benefits of intoxication are necessary to shed light on his ambivalence and balance the apparent commitment to 'healing love'.

At this point, it is unclear whether Rupert has the will and inner resources to recognize and challenge his attachment to substance use and users. He appears to be in crisis at the moment and this is a time of both opportunity and threat. On the one hand, he has organized counselling for himself, thus taking action on his wish to free himself of the hold of his past, and patterns around mood altering substances are an aspect of this. He is identifying his feelings about his partner and manager and is currently sustaining both those relationships. On the other hand, he appears to be reactive in the face of change, rather than proactive, and perhaps somewhat identified with the roles of victim and rescuer as in the Transactional

Analysis (TA) drama triangle. Does he have issues about anger, perhaps? How willing and able is he to face this discomfort and address his need for an intoxicated partner?

What it might take to approach and resolve, at least partially, these substance-related issues cannot be ascertained until Rupert has clarified his own wants and priorities. In the shorter term, possible avenues to follow include developing conflict management skills to help him in his relationships at work, exploring the significance of his marijuana use through a diary of cues and consequences, discovering alternative ways of managing anxiety and anger and looking in more detail at Rupert's discomfort with his partner. By enabling Rupert to examine his expectations, hopes and fears about his partner's 'recovery' versus what is actually happening, and by identifying realistic alternatives to withdrawal, it may be possible for the two of them to survive the changes together and even benefit from them. In the longer term, Rupert probably needs space for his inner child, and to learn to direct some of his love inwards to heal himself. However, the deeper levels of work cannot be tackled effectively whilst he remains overwhelmed with the present crises in his life or if he is retreating into intoxication.

The need to consider whether the client's substance use and sexual preferences are interrelated or not

Never assume there is a relationship between a client's problematic use of mood altering drugs and sexual orientation. In some instances it could be direct and clear, as in the case of the happily married man who periodically gets very drunk and engages in anonymous sex with other men and hates himself for it. For others, there may be no connection other than, say, a hesitation to trust a psychotherapist to be accepting and comfortable with the client's lifestyle.

It is important for us as practitioners not to delude ourselves into thinking we can hide our views and reactions from clients. Clients are often sensitive to the subtle – and not so subtle – forms in which people give away their true stance, be this through body language, voice tone, use of language or choices and omissions in our interventions.

It may be valuable to consider language in more depth at this point, as this is a confusing area in various subcultures of both sexual orientation and substance use. Imagine that a client says to you: 'Do you think I'm an alcoholic faggot because I never dared stand up to my father?' What assumptions might you make about the meaning and purpose of his question? *Consider how you might respond to this question before reading on.*

Is this client expressing his belief or felt-sense of the interconnections between his denial and sexual orientation as expressions of his terror of being himself? Is he expressing self-hatred of the child that he was, or perhaps testing whether he may express anger at his father with you? Is he assessing your attitude to his drinking and/or his sexual orientation? Does he wear the label 'alcoholic' to mark his positive identification with the disease concept of drink-related difficulties and the fellowship of Alcoholics Anonymous, or is it a term imbued with shame and confusion? Is he part of a group engaged in 'queer politics', which has an active commitment to destigmatize words such as 'faggot' and challenge a society threatened by diversity? Is he encouraging you to set yourself up on a pedestal of expertise, so he can watch you topple and avoid considering self-change? Or is there an entirely different purpose to the question?

Think back to the response you identified above. Would it enable the client to explore openly and comfortably what he meant or did you implicitly or explicitly direct him according to your interests?

The distinction between listening with empathy and listening with response

As far as possible, do not use the client to work through your own issues. Be prepared to create the support and challenge you need outside your relationship with the client to explore your own patterns of substance use. Consider what myths and values you hold and what your assumptions, fantasies and reactions tell you about *you*. Be non-defensive and develop a moment by moment awareness of when your capacity to listen to the client with empathy is obscured by your listening with response. These responses may be related in more or less direct ways to substance use and/or sexual orientations and lifestyles.

To grasp this principle more deeply, try the following 'trigger comments' exercise, ideally in a group so you can compare responses. Imagine one of your clients making the first of the statements below and consider what your gut reaction would be. We suggest you make a note of what feelings and judgements arise for you. Next, think about the precise wording of an empathic response to this client and write this down. Finally, consider and note what issues are raised for you that you may need to explore further, given the difference, if any, between your gut reaction and empathic response. Then proceed similarly with the next statement and so on through the list.

Woman: Ever since we decided to have a child and have been practising self-insemination, I'm sure Marie is smoking crack again.
Man: I'm really happy with Bob, even though he's old enough to be my father. But I really think he's drinking too much and I've not dared go for help 'cos we could get into trouble, me being only 17.
Bisexual woman: It's when I'm stoned, I just forget about safer sex... Sometimes I even forget that I have HIV.
Woman: I finally told Mum I was a lesbian and do you know what she

said? She said, whatever you do, don't tell your father, it'll kill him. No wonder I used on top of my script this week.

To counsellor of the same sex: I'm embarrassed about this and I bet it happens to you all the time, but since I got clean . . . I don't think it's the counselling I'm coming for . . .

Woman: There's definitely something going on between me and Sarah. But it only happens after raves and we never talk about it at other times.

Man: Errol's back into Special Brew in a big way. Says he just can't cut it in a man's body.

The need to assess dependency and harm

Take the time to develop the knowledge base described above. Learn how to assess dependency and harm. This is a crucial aspect of general assessment and as vital to the client's well-being as knowledge of mental health problems, being able to recognize which clients may be at risk of self-harm, which may have been sexually abused and so on. Consider for instance whether it is ethical to ignore, through ignorance or neglect, the signs of chemical dependency and physical damage, in the way you work with a client?

The typical lack of awareness within the psychotherapy and counselling professions, as in the general public, of the nature and consequences of different levels of alcohol and drug use and the abundant myths which often serve to obscure awareness of our own patterns of substance use, contribute to the mistreatment of lesbians, gay and bisexual people.

Case example 2

Consider the following example. Had you been Hope's counsellor, what might have alerted you to the real nature of her problem?

> Ever since her ex-lover suddenly died Hope had been finding it increasingly difficult to leave her flat, particularly during the day. Finally, she decided to consult a counsellor. They spent several months exploring her feelings about being bisexual, her fears of death, the dynamics of her childhood and her relationship with her previous partners. Although she valued the deeper self-awareness this gave her, the acute anxiety she felt when going out did not abate. Through her GP, she was referred to a psychologist with whom she worked cognitively and behaviourally on her 'agoraphobia' and 'panic attacks'. After several sessions, Hope became terrified that this psychologist was condemning her because she was a lesbian and broke off the relationship. She became increasingly despondent and felt more and more suicidal.
>
> A supportive ex-lover invited her to visit him in the States, where she stayed out on a farm. For several days, she suffered acute anxiety, where she found herself shaking uncontrollably, could not eat, found

her sleep fitful with night sweats and terrible nightmares. Hope became convinced she was seriously ill and prepared to return to England, only she could not face the journey. Then, after a week she began to feel much better, more relaxed and started to sleep soundly. Delighted but unable to understand the reasons for her increasing physical and emotional well-being, Hope returned to England and began to work as a volunteer in a charity.

It was through a chance discussion with another volunteer, who himself had been drink dependent, that Hope realized her anxiety had actually been a physical symptom of alcohol withdrawal. She had been drinking about two bottles of wine every evening prior to her trip to the USA, but wrongly attributed all her feelings of panic and depression to her psychological state and none of the professionals working with her had considered physical causes. She was fortunate that she had not been prescribed tranquillizers for depression for, whilst they would have removed the anxiety symptoms, they would have potentiated the alcohol, having a similar effect on the brain and central nervous system, making withdrawal much more severe and dangerous. Hope was also fortunate not to have had a professional urge her to cut down on her drinking, for this would have probably led to an intolerable increase in her withdrawal symptoms, causing her to drink more and feel guilty and ashamed, making her self-esteem plummet further.

The importance of exploring the benefits and costs of the client's present lifestyle

Remember that every lifestyle has its advantages as well as disadvantages and that behaviour that persists must be perceived as valuable to the person in some way. Do not take sides in an inner conflict within a client, other than by demonstrating your trust in their essential wisdom. The client may initially try to persuade you to align yourself with their 'critical parent' and if you are tempted to tell them what is wrong with their way of life, they may privately become more identified with the advantages of that lifestyle, and be less likely to want to change.

Case example 3
Look at this example and think about what you may consider to be the benefits and costs of Morgan's lifestyle as it changes.

> Morgan spent his youth running away from children's homes and short term foster placements, mainly in white families. He survived by offering sex in return for accommodation and developed a cocaine habit. In his early 20s, he found a sense of self-identity and racial

pride through Islam, and managed to overcome his craving for cocaine. His marriage lasted four years before Morgan attempted suicide, unable to deal with the growing pressures his impotence was causing. The crisis left Morgan estranged from his community and very confused about his identity. He moved to another city, found work and a place to live, but felt very isolated and began to drink heavily. His health suffered and when he was diagnosed with a peptic ulcer, his doctor referred him to an alcohol counsellor. With support, Morgan managed three months largely alcohol free and began to consider whether he was gay, but could not bring himself to discuss this with his counsellor and stopped attending. When he finally plucked up the courage to visit the local gay bar, he found himself unable to bear the way he felt treated as an exotic specimen and began to drink again. He developed a reputation for erratic violence and was barred from clubs and pubs in his locality.

The next crisis occurred when he lost his job and was evicted from his flat for non-payment of rent. After a period of sleeping rough, he was resettled through a local charity on condition he attended AA meetings. Once more he felt completely isolated and doubly oppressed as black and possibly gay. He was recommended to attend a gay AA meeting but panicked when he was sexually approached by a couple of group members and never went back.

Whilst Morgan found the courage and will despite the odds, to maintain abstinence for weeks at a time, periodically he 'went on a bender' and drank heavily for days. After several periods of hospitalization, Morgan developed a therapeutic relationship with an alcohol counsellor and they worked together for two years on harm reduction. At the end of this time, he was still bout drinking and at other times 'cottaging' . However, he had organized his life to minimize the dangers and also the frequency of his 'lapses' from sexual and alcohol abstinence, which were the goals he ultimately chose for himself.

Awareness of the stages of change

Remind yourself regularly, especially if you experience impatience, frustration or despair in relation to your clients, just how hard it is to change a well-established and ingrained way of life. Consider the stages of change and what the client may need to work through as well as where they are now in the process of change. It is sometimes useful to remember how you approach and negotiate change.

You may find it useful to consider integrative and 'transtheoretical' approaches to working with change (Prochaska and Di Clemente 1983) as they provide guidelines to help you identify stages in the process and to choose appropriate interventions for that stage. The example of Morgan above illustrates the many levels at which a client may need to consider and address life issues. Change at these levels is neither uniform nor linear and as therapists, we need to be flexible, accepting, patient and highly sensitive to the current needs, priorities and resources of our clients.

Conclusions

- It is very tempting for therapists to avoid working with people who are struggling with issues that distress or perplex us. We may do this by referring them on to 'specialists', having decided they are inappropriate for the service we offer. We may deny the nature of the issues with which they are struggling, and label them 'difficult', 'unmotivated' or 'resistant', or we may insist they deal with those issues that excite us.
- Although the ethical principles of competence, responsibility and integrity can never be fully realized, a commitment to humility, non-defensiveness and good practice can go a long way towards facilitating a more satisfactory lifestyle for clients such as those described above. Making good use of supervision and additional training can also bring enormous benefits to this work.
- *Everyone* is a potential user of mood-changing substances.
- Anyone can experience problems connected with their own, or another's, substance use.
- Substance use is widespread in all cultures and subcultures, and takes many forms – depressants, narcotic analgesics, stimulants and hallucinogens.
- Alcohol is the drug causing greatest damage, yet it is the most socially acceptable.
- There is no one 'true way' to deal with problems with substance use, or a single correct framework to describe its complexities.
- Lesbians and gay men report more problems with substance use, a higher rate of use and a longer 'career' of using than heterosexuals, yet form a lower proportion of those benefiting from appropriate professional help.
- To witness the capacity of the human spirit to overcome difficulties and flourish against all the odds is perhaps the most inspiring and rewarding experience our professional lives can offer us. That capacity is eminently discernible in those clients we have met, who are struggling with issues of sexual orientation and substance use.

12 | FRAN WALSH

Partner abuse

> Then I got pushed up against the door frame and was getting punched and kicked in the crotch. It really freaked me out, here I was being held and battered, and there was nothing I could do. Then I got thrown to the ground, and she was on top of me banging my head on the floor.

If you had read this extract out of the context of this chapter, you may have been surprised that the perpetrator turned out to be a woman. You may have been even more surprised to learn that the person being attacked was the woman she professed to love and with whom she had been in a relationship for some four years.

Over the past few years poster campaigns, television talk shows and even soap operas have ensured that the term 'domestic violence' has become a familiar phrase. However, it is generally understood to be a heterosexual problem. Although there have been few studies into domestic violence in same sex relationships, those which do exist, coupled with much anecdotal evidence, suggest that the problem can be found in *all* types of intimate relationship.

In this chapter, I propose to explore the issue of same sex partner abuse – what it is, the similarities and differences to heterosexual partner abuse, and the ways in which we, as therapists, can respond. Most counselling and therapeutic training offered at present spends little or no time dealing with the problems of working with clients involved in abusive relationships. This general lack of expertise is often compounded for many therapists by a lack of understanding of the specific issues encountered when working with lesbian or gay clients. I will address some of the issues which you may need to think about as therapists working with lesbian or gay clients, some of whom may indeed be involved in relationships which could be defined as abusive.

For the purposes of this chapter I will be using the term 'partner abuse' as opposed to 'domestic violence'. The reason for this is that, while domestic violence is a term often used to describe abuses which take place in a wide variety of relationships, for many people it still conjures up an image of heterosexual home and family situations. Also, the word 'violence' can create an expectation about the type of abuse which may be taking place. This can result in the therapist holding an hierarchy of abuse where physical violence is more important, and therefore more of an issue than emotional or psychological abuse. Rather than stretching the phrase 'domestic violence' to encompass all the possible types of relationships and of abuses which may occur within them, I have chosen the phrase 'partner abuse'. This offers a more wide ranging definition of the issues which we will be exploring.

It is also important to note than when I refer to same sex relationships, I am including relationships where one, or both parties, may define themselves as bisexual but who are at present in a same sex relationship.

What is partner abuse?

Farley (1992) defines partner abuse as acts of psychological or physical aggression in which the perpetrator attempts to intimidate or harm another within an intimate relationship. Partner abuse can take a number of forms, or a combination of many, such as:

- constant criticism;
- threats;
- insults;
- being slapped, kicked or punched;
- things being thrown at someone;
- attack with a weapon;
- injury with a weapon;
- inflicting cuts, bruises or broken bones;
- being humiliated;
- rape;
- murder.

Partner abuse is an area where myths abound; it is important that we recognize their existence and impact in our own practices as therapists and on our clients' attitudes to their own difficulties. A few of the most common myths are:

Myth: Some people ask for it.
Reality: It will often be the case that the abusive partner will justify violent or abusive behaviour as being the result of some provocation from their partner. However, it is an important starting point when working with this issue to recognize that abuse (whether physical or psychological) in a relationship is never an appropriate or acceptable way of dealing with any situation. No one ever asks to be abused; whatever the dynamics of

the situation, the responsibility for the abusive behaviour always lies with the abuser.

Myth: If it's not physical then it's not as bad.

Reality: Abuse does not have to be physical to have an impact. To be constantly criticized, verbally abused or humiliated can leave someone with the same strength and variety of emotions as if they had been hospitalized by their partner's actions. Many survivors of partner abuse will say that it was the psychological abuse that was more damaging and took longer to recover from.

Myth: It is caused by drink or drugs.

Reality: It is a common belief that drink or drugs are always the root cause of abusive behaviour. While they may be a trigger to this kind of behaviour, they can by no means offer a full explanation of the problem. Not everyone who drinks or uses drugs is abusive and not everyone who abuses their partner is either drunk or using drugs.

Myth: It's only a working-class problem.

Reality: Even today, images of drunken, uneducated, working-class people living in poor housing, and regularly battering each other senseless may come to mind when we hear about violent relationships. However, partner abuse is a problem which occurs across all classes and cultures. It is important to us as therapists to realize that our highly educated, articulate and charming middle-class client may just as easily be a perpetrator or recipient of partner abuse.

Myth: They could just leave.

Reality: For many people living in a situation of partner abuse, leaving may sound like an obvious solution. However, it may be more difficult than it seems for a number of reasons. They may believe that their partner loves them and that the behaviour will change and things will get better. They may have nowhere to go. It is not unusual for the abuser to damage their partner's confidence to the extent that they do not maintain relationships outside of the partnership, and do not have the strength or confidence to leave without support. They may be financially or practically tied to their partner, e.g. owning a house or running a business together. Or they may just feel the abuse is something that they deserve and should or can put up with.

Myth: Abuse is perpetrated by men against female partners.

Reality: Partner abuse is perpetrated by men and women within same sex, and different sex, relationships. It is important for therapists to acknowledge that women in heterosexual relationships also abuse male partners.

Partner abuse can take place in any relationship and can take many forms. As therapists we must be careful not to allow our own attitudes to the problem to blind us to its presence in the lives of our clients.

Same sex partner abuse: comparisons with the heterosexual problem

One of the major pitfalls facing therapists working with clients involved in abusive same sex relationships is to approach it from a position which assumes that it is just like working with heterosexual clients. This is a misconception. Offering appropriate, high quality therapy to gay men and lesbians in this situation is dependent on an understanding of both the similarities and the differences.

Gender

In cross-gender relationships it is an 'accepted wisdom' that the relative power imbalance (physical, cultural, economic) between men and women has an effect on partner abuse, both in the roots of the violence and in the capacity of women to respond or extricate themselves from the situation. By far the majority of reported cases of partner abuse come from women physically abused by men.

Power imbalances arising from gender expectations will not be present within a same sex relationship. This can lead to a number of problems. Often it makes it harder for those viewing the relationship from the outside to identify the 'real victim'. It may be easier to understand how a woman can be abused, terrorized and intimidated by her male partner to the extent that she feels unable to challenge the behaviour or leave the relationship. In same sex relationships however, what we might assume we see are two people ostensibly physically and socially matched in terms of power, one of whom is abusing the other. The danger of this is that those working with a person who is experiencing abuse at the hands of a same sex partner may well trivialize or underestimate the seriousness of the situation, writing it off as merely an argument or a fight. This can compound the client's sense that this is not really abuse or that they should have been able to fight back, leave, change the situation, or never have allowed it to happen in the first place. In the case of the abuser this attitude can confirm their belief that there has been no abuse and that their partner is at least as culpable for what has happened. This may be doubly compounded for gay men, who will be struggling with an abusive situation in the context of their own masculinity in our culture.

Case example 1
J certainly believes that, as a man, he should have been more able to stop the abuse that he experienced in his relationship of two years:

> I don't understand what happened to me. I never thought I'd be in a situation like that, well it happens to other people, women you know, not a man like me. I know that if I told people they'd just think, 'Why

didn't he stop it? He's a big bloke.' I don't know why I didn't, I just know I felt like I couldn't.

J is himself a victim of fixed expectations of masculinity and male roles within relationships. Lesbians and gay men in relationships are having always to deconstruct, or struggle to maintain, or rebel against internalized gender and role expectations which need reframing in relation to two people of the same gender being partners. It is imperative that the therapist is able to reframe these expectations for themselves and with their client. Men, in general, are known to underreport abuse against themselves.

It is true that there is not a gender imbalance with all its cultural implications, in a same sex relationship. Nevertheless there can clearly be, in any relationship, a power imbalance based on the dynamics existing between the couple, the relative personal power wielded by each partner as well as economic and physical strength differentials.

The similarities

Like their heterosexual counterparts, lesbians and gay men who are subjected to partner abuse can experience any combination of a range of physical, sexual and psychological abuse. The type of abuse inflicted by same sex partners can be just as inventive and damaging as that inflicted by heterosexuals.

Often the responses of the abused partner and the abuser in same sex relationships will share a great number of similarities to those expressed by heterosexual couples. Lesbian and gay survivors may well trivialize and understate their experiences. They may blame themselves or try to justify the abuser's behaviour and insist that they can help the abuser to change.

Case example 2

C had been in a relationship for some months before it began to deteriorate. Eventually her partner began to physically attack C. C's response, in one particularly violent incident where she was kicked and punched after a party, was to look at her own behaviour for a trigger to the assault. 'I think that she wouldn't have done it if I'd taken more notice of her; you see there were a lot of my friends there and she felt I hadn't given her enough attention. She's really insecure. I should have known that.'

Like their heterosexual counterparts, abused partners may well find themselves to be isolated and trapped, not only by their own situation, but also by a lack of outside recognition and support. Abusers will often deny responsibility, blaming their partner or the situation for the abuse. Sometimes they will deny point-blank that their behaviour is, in fact, abusive.

Despite these similarities, there are a number of very significant differences which are present in the case of same sex partner abuse which will have an impact on our work as therapists with clients in this situation.

The differences

Homophobia

Homophobia is the major experiential difference (see Chapter 3). Homophobia will almost certainly figure as an extra difficulty having impact on same sex partner abuse. External homophobia – that is, prejudice emanating from outside sources – may well affect the abuse situation in a number of ways. For the abused partner it may limit their access to outside support, e.g. advice agencies, the police, support groups, even therapists. In a culture where being lesbian or gay at all can be a reason to be sacked, discriminated against and generally disapproved of, to come out as a recipient of same sex partner abuse must be doubly difficult. Add to this the inexperience, prejudice or lack of gay awareness training of many of the helping or legal agencies and the fact that 'queer bashing' is, arguably, culturally reinforced.

As with external homophobia, the individual's own 'internalized homophobia' (defined in Chapter 3) may well have impact on both the abused and the abuser. For the abuser it may form part of a low self-image which they seek to bolster up by having, and exerting, power over their partner. It may also be that their partner embodies some of the elements of their own sexual identity that the abuser feels unhappy about. For instance, if the partner is a camp gay man, this may be an expression of gay identity which, deep down, is distasteful to his lover to the point that the lover becomes persecutory. This does not make the abuse the fault of the abused partner. Rather, it is the problem of the abuser precipitated by his internalized homophobia.

For those partners in a relationship who are being abused, their internalized homophobia can cause them to feel like the relationship is in itself wrong – a manifestation of their own 'sick sexuality'. As such, it is not difficult to understand that the abused partner may see the abuse as just another aspect of an already 'perverted' relationship.

Some other areas may require special consideration in the context of same sex partner abuse.

Sado-masochism

Having to define and redefine their relationship to prescribed gender and social roles, lesbians and gay men tend to be more open about consensual sado-masochistic practices and it is therefore likely that anyone working with these groups will at some point come across this. It is important in such a situation not to confuse S&M practices with any form of abuse and for the therapist to be clear that, as long as both parties are in agreement as to the type, severity and expression of such acts, then there is no abuse involved.

It may, however, be the case that one or other partner is not happy with the activities, or feels that things are going too far. It would then be useful to help your client to identify how they want to change things and negotiate boundaries and agreements which suit them. It is important that you try to have as clear an understanding as possible about the issues and practices of S&M sexuality. If your client is aware of judgemental or negative attitudes on your part, this could lead to alienation and damage the therapeutic relationship.

Rape and sexual assault
It is important to recognize that both lesbians and gay men are capable of being sexually assaulted, or of sexually assaulting others.

In the law, rape is now defined as unlawful sexual intercourse with someone who, at the time, does not give consent to it. The Criminal Justice Act of 1994 provided for the prosecution of men who have 'unlawful intercourse' with other men and several cases since have led to conviction. Sexual assault is called *indecent assault* and can refer to a physical or non-physical assault. Definitions of rape are very specific and deal with the concept of penile penetration. As such, they may not be wide enough to encompass all experiences of 'rape' in the non-legal sense. Therapists need to accept the client's definition of the assault which has happened. Many men and women who have been sexually assaulted by their same sex partners will describe what has happened to them as rape, thus defining the impact of the experience. As with physical and emotional abuse, survivors of sexual attack by same sex partners (or strangers) will express many responses in common with their heterosexual counterparts. Feelings of shame, anger, guilt, shock, terror, grief or self-blame may all be present. However, for those assaulted by a member of the same sex there may well be a number of other feelings present. For men it is often very difficult to come to terms with having been raped. We live in a society where men are expected to be able to protect themselves, indeed it is generally believed that men are the sexual aggressors in our culture, not the victims. There are particular cultural stigmas at work around masculinity and penetration.

Women may have difficulty in acknowledging the assault as rape, while still experiencing the powerful impact of the assault 'as if it were a real rape'. As K said,

> One of the most important bits of the counselling for me was when I was able to call what she did to me 'rape'. It opened up the floodgates

and at last I was able to sort out some of my feelings around it. I don't feel like I'm overreacting now.

Women in this situation need support in validating their own experience of the assault regardless of the legal definitions of the attack. Women who do acknowledge the impact of the assault may also have to face the enormous sense of disappointment and disillusionment at having been sexually assaulted by another woman.

An important facet of gay affirmative therapy is a sensitivity to feelings of shame and disappointment experienced by some lesbians and gay men when their relationships become damaged or abusive. This may involve the loss of a dream that gay would turn out better than straight, or fighting off negative messages about the 'inevitable' failures of same sex relationships (see Chapter 6) and possibly a reluctance, as a result, to disclose problems to others.

Co-battery
When there is similarity in the physical capacities of partners in a same sex relationship it is not uncommon for a person being physically abused by their partner to hit back eventually. This can sometimes lead to confusion about who abused whom and who the 'real victim' is. As therapists, it is part of our role to help the client to clarify the situation.

> The message that we want to impart is that self protection is not co-battery, whether [s/he] strikes back at the time of the battery or at some other time. And although occasionally using more force than is necessary to defend her [him] self may be something [s/he] wishes to avoid, it hardly qualifies as abuse.
> (Burstow 1992: 171)

Implications for therapists

Having looked at some issues which may arise in relation to same sex abuse it is important now to explore some of the implications for both the therapy and the therapist. Probably the most important first consideration for any therapist working, or planning to work, with a client involved in an abusive same sex relationship is to be clear about your own limitations. If there are any reasons at all why you may feel that your value systems or beliefs might make it difficult for you to offer an open and respectful relationship to your client, which is affirming of their lifestyle choices, then it is important that you decide not to work with this person. If, for example, you were unable to accept a client's decision to stay in an abusive relationship then it would not be beneficial to them to continue working with you. Instead, it would be better for you to offer some alternative referral to a therapist whom you believe to be able to offer appropriate therapy.

When writing about lesbian victims of relationship abuse, Nancy Hammond (1989: 97) says:

> A lesbian battering or abuse victim seeking emotional support from mainstream counsellors and mental health providers faces all the risks of coming out... In addition she enters into a relationship that can be expected to involve extended contact over time in a context that promotes added emotional vulnerability. In these circumstances the sensitivity with which the counsellor or therapist approaches both domestic violence and sexual preference issues will be critical in restoring the victim's sense of well being.

It is no less true for gay men embarking on therapy that the respect with which the therapist approaches these issues will have an impact on the client's sense of self-worth and validity.

The maintenance of a respectful approach involves a number of specific considerations for therapists working with lesbian and gay clients in abusive relationships.

Taking the situation seriously

As we have seen previously in this chapter, it can sometimes be hard enough for a person experiencing abuse to take it seriously for themselves. It is therefore often helpful if someone outside the relationship can make it clear that they recognize the seriousness of the situation. It is imperative that you do not underestimate the kind of danger which may be present in an abusive relationship, even when the client herself or himself may be denying that danger. Labelling abusive behaviours as such will, in itself, be of great significance.

Challenging trivialization, denial or self-blame

Part of taking the situation seriously involves challenging trivialization, denial or self-blame on the part of the client. It is important to show your client that, while you can empathize with their experience of the situation, you do not collude with the client's trivialization, denial or self-blame. For instance, if a client who is persistently coming to therapy bruised and cut insists that 'this is nothing – we just had a fight', the therapist can find a way of feeding back their own perceptions of the situation, perhaps by pointing out the extent of the injuries or the frequency of the fights. This kind of challenge to the client's perception must be done very carefully and with a great deal of respect for the client. Nothing can be as damaging to a relationship as a therapist who insists that their reality take precedence over that of the client. The client has a right to hold on to their version of the truth, but it need not be the therapist's.

Empowering clients

It is always up to the individual whether they choose to stay in, or leave, a relationship. However, the therapist can be instrumental in helping the client to explore all the options. As part of this process of empowerment, it may be useful for the therapist to be able to offer information about services or networks available to support the client. Empowering the client does not mean encouraging them to leave the relationship. Leaving in itself does not always make someone safe from the abuse. Some people are abused by ex-partners and the point at which a relationship is being dissolved can often be the most dangerous in terms of escalation of abuse. A key aim of therapy is to increase awareness and choice within a framework of realism.

Working with abusers

There is much debate as to the best way to work with abusers. There can be little doubt that it is particularly useful for abusers to work in a group setting. Here, issues such as anger management, accountability and focusing on stopping the abusive behaviour can be confronted with, and by, others who have been in a similar role in their own relationships.

However, such groups are often hard enough to come by for those in heterosexual relationships. For gay men and lesbians who are involved in abusing their partners, it is almost impossible (see, however, agencies in Appendix 2). Left then with the only option being individual therapy, it is obviously the responsibility of the therapist not to collude with the client's denial or refusal to accept responsibility for their actions. As with working with survivors the therapist must use their challenging skills to avoid such a collusion.

Couples counselling

On the whole, couples counselling is not considered to be the best form of therapy for those involved in abusive relationships. There are a number of reasons for this. It is impossible to ensure the safety of the abused partner; it would be possible, for instance, for the abuser to use disclosures made during the therapy as vehicles for further abuse. Also, if a considerable amount of individual work has not been done, it is easy for the therapy sessions to mirror the dynamics already present in the relationship, thus confirming a sense of inevitability and powerlessness on the part of the abused partner, and 'right' on that of the abuser.

Susan L. Morrow and Donna Hawxhurst (1989: 61), in their piece on working with lesbian partner abuse, say of couples counselling:

> If after extensive [individual] work the couple wishes to reunite, counselling should be done by a therapist who is cognisant of the battering history and is familiar with battering dynamics. It should be the survivor, not the batterer or the counsellor, who initiates readiness for couples counselling.

Conclusions

- Partner abuse can occur in any relationship and takes a wide range of forms.
- Partner abuse is not restricted by class, status, race, gender, size, economics, education or sexuality. Complex and subtle power imbalances may be involved.
- Responsibility for abuse always lies with the perpetrator.
- Psychological or emotional abuse is no less damaging than physical kinds.
- Alcohol and drugs are not always a causal factor.
- There are many similarities between cross-gender and same sex partner abuse and some important differences for therapists to take into account. These include differences of gender and role expectations, the experiences arising from homophobia and its internalization and the higher frequencies of sado-masochistic sexual practices in same sex relationships.
- Therapists need to accept and work with clients' own definitions of rape and sexual assaults and to be aware of the different issues arising for men, for women and for those in same sex relationships in which these assaults occur.
- Therapists need to challenge trivialization by clients (or in themselves) of abusive behaviours as well as denial and self-blame and to focus on empowerment and choice. Group work is more successful with abusers, though hard to find, and couples therapy is not recommended where partner abuse is happening.
- Resources are listed in the Appendixes.

13 BERNARD LYNCH

Religious and spirituality conflicts

Psychotherapy and spirituality are closely related. When we recognize the origins of the term 'healing the soul' (or psyche), we can construct an authentic psychotherapeutic approach. In my quest for understanding the sources of people's pain and its cures, I must affirm on the most profound level that wholeness, holiness and fullness of life can come to the individual through an understanding of God in their life. This approach I call psychospiritual growth.

This chapter offers a non-technical sketch of a theology of healing and personal integration, or psychospirituality, which is applied practically in working with those in conflict with their religion or their spiritual development. I will contend that the impact of organized Christian religions on the psychological and spiritual well-being of lesbians, gay men and bisexual men and women has been negative at best and frequently extremely destructive. It will be helpful to begin with a shared understanding of some key terms. It is important to distinguish between religious and spiritual experience.

Spiritual experience transcends our everyday experience of ourselves in the world. It offers insight into, or connection with, the existence of something more profound. These occurrences cannot be explained easily because our language is rooted in everyday life, but an important part of working psychospiritually involves therapist and client constructing together language, symbols and metaphors with which to communicate their meaning. Spiritual experience is engagement with God in ourselves. Organized religions have, in a sense, interrupted the direct relationship between ourselves and God in ourselves and attempted to own or control that spiritual link. Over history, mainstream religions such as Christianity and Islam have taken over spiritual experience and applied their own meaning to it, often also imposing a political agenda. In this way religious institutions act as powerful agents of social control imposing moral authority, often on the basis of selective scriptural interpretation. *Religious experience*, then, will be a person's experience of the church's place, significance, meanings and teachings in their life, the history and relationships they have had with the church.

Mainstream churches do not affirm diverse sexualities in terms of lifestyle or spirituality. From Biblical fundamentalism to Roman dogmatism, lesbian, gay and bisexual people have been ostracized and persecuted. At the same time, and increasingly, there are real attempts to separate this oppression from a spiritual quest for meaning: a search for God.

Christianity and homosexuality

No mainstream churches accept homosexuality as a valid and healthy expression of the self, with the notable exception of the Society of Friends (Quakers). Nor are lesbians and gay men's needs catered for in any of the churches' rituals or services (Boswell 1980, 1989, 1994 gives historical exceptions). In fact, we go almost wholly unrecognized, the validity of our being is denied and our lifestyles condemned. At best we are tolerated within a 'love the sinner, hate the sin' framework.

In 1986, the infamous 'Halloween Letter' from Cardinal Ratzinger's office at the Vatican (formerly the Holy Office of the Inquisition!) boldly stated that, 'Homosexuals are disordered in their nature and evil in their love'; not very different from the Prophet Mohammed's view that 'Allah has cursed him who indulges in this evil act of the people of Lut' (Haddith: An-Nasa'i, quoted in Thompson 1993). This most basic denial of homosexual experience makes it difficult to imagine finding spiritual guidance or development from these sources.

Christianity, as manifested in the teachings and practices of its major churches, has difficulties dealing with sexuality generally. At the heart of the faith is the belief in an incarnate God – a God who became flesh. Yet the churches promote a process of disincarnation and disembodiment. Religious authenticity and human authenticity are one. It is not what we say about God that ultimately matters but who we are as a result of our belief in that God. Are we more free? Are we more human? As Saint Iraneus put it in the third century, 'Gloria Dei Vivans Homo': the glory of God is woman/man fully alive.

Judaism and Islam, which share the same fundamental roots as Christianity, offer neither in their orthodoxy nor their praxis positive models of lesbian and gay spirituality. Eastern religions seem similarly intolerant on the whole and sex is rarely mentioned, except within the dialectics of marriage and family.

Sexuality is about relationality; it is not simply a question of whom one chooses to go to bed with or what one does there although, naturally, it may include this. Sexuality has as much to do with how we appreciate music, participate in athletics or celebrate mass as it has to do with our love-making; it is our selfhood being expressed. One cannot underestimate the negative effect of religion in the lives of lesbian and gay people brought up in a particular tradition. Merely offering a humanist alternative is not adequate as it does not necessarily address the person's spiritual needs. The whole process of spiritual and religious learning needs working through with the client and mutually redefining.

Case example 1
Immediately upon entering therapy John presented the Sodom and Gomorrah story (Genesis 19: 4–11) and St Paul's epistle to the Romans (Chapter 1: 26) as reasons as to why he could not be gay. After referring him to some readings (e.g. Fortunato 1982; McNeill 1988; Glaser 1990; see Appendix 3), which enabled him to understand that there are other scholarly ways of interpreting these passages, I was able to help him move into what was important for him in terms of his relationship to the God, the Christ, and how he could integrate this into his own sexual-relational life.

For many people such as John the presenting problem is first and foremost one of education or indoctrination around what I have come to call 'Bible bingo'. This is the selective and destructive use of Biblical (or Talmudic or Koranic) passages to back arguments for a patriarchal, heterosexist and homophobic world view. At the same time, the historical and cultural contexts of other passages (e.g. 'God created the world in six days') are completely glossed over. (Bibliotherapy is discussed further in Chapter 3.)

It is not unusual to meet people in therapy who have been psychosexually mutilated by their religious background. They have had the seed of their relationality almost removed. Is it any wonder that the suicide rate is so high among young gay people, as we saw in Chapter 8? We only see those whose pain, or courage, has forced them to our consulting rooms. The damage to their humanity and self-valuing is often pathological.

All the main religions I know condemn young people who are not heterosexual to a never ending sexual carousel because they 'forgive' sexual activity while discouraging and denying same sex sexual loving. In denying lesbians, gay men and bisexuals their intrinsic goodness, the churches deny them their godliness. Self-alienation is God alienation: 'In this breakthrough I discover that God and I are one', says Meister Eckhart (quoted in Fox 1983: 120). Coming to terms with the self is coming to terms with God in ourselves. Who we are as whole human beings is what ultimately bespeaks our expression of God.

When the client presents with religious issues the demythologizing that must be done will demand of the therapist clear perceptions of what is religious, cultural and historical and what is more deeply spiritual. Any confusion between these can be detrimental to the client. Supervision is imperative in this process. As the client gets deeper into psychospiritual issues and closer to themselves, they may become alienated from their broader communities – religious, familial, cultural. This experience can be the conduit to a transference of deep anger and resentment towards the therapist. Anger is often necessary if the client is to move into their authenticity and freedom; from this space wholeness and holiness can grow. We saw in Chapter 2 the profound importance of working through grief and anger resulting from the internalizing of oppression if genuine healing is to occur.

Lesbian and gay spirituality: ritual and ceremony

We have said the churches deny validation of lesbian and gay life experiences and access to ritualistic expression of spirituality. There is no marriage, even if wanted, nor any service of commitment. Partners may be buried by the church but generally there is no formal recognition of the grief of the remaining partner nor comfort from the institutionalized God within the church's rites. Same sex love threatens the system of church control over relationality.

In the past, the response of lesbians and gay men has been to tend their wounds, limping away from the oppression of Christianity in particular and religion in general. However, the onslaught of AIDS has compelled us to fight for the right to rituals and ceremonies marking significant events in our lives, and to reclaim and reassert a spirituality related directly to same sex love. Most do not want merely to ape heterosexist religious orthodoxy but seek to create forms unique to their lives and lifestyles. Dignity in the USA, the Metropolitan Community Church, the Lesbian and Gay Christian Movement and Quest in the UK are excellent examples of where this is happening (see Appendix 2). The works of John McNeil and Elizabeth Stewart provide a much needed discourse in which to debate new thinking (see Appendix 3).

Case example 2
Charlie and David are one example among many of my experience in this area. I met them while vacationing in Spain in 1984. Over the years, on trips back and forth from New York, we stayed in touch and became friends. During this time I learned that both were HIV positive.

In the autumn of 1991, in London for a conference, I telephoned their home to see how they were doing. David was dying. Charlie asked me to come to their flat, saying that if I could 'do something' they would be very grateful. Neither Charlie nor David had, to my knowledge, any formal religious background. In fact, when I respectfully asked what I could do, David had requested Charlie to ask me to bring 'the Eucalyptus' (Eucharist!). Together we created a secular service on themes of love, life and death. A non-religious, deeply spiritual ceremony is commonly requested of someone in my profession in the AIDS pandemic. David died peacefully in Charlie's arms that evening.

Subsequently, I was asked to take David's funeral service and provide once more 'something' which would speak to a non-religious group of Charlie's and David's families and friends. Several days later Charlie said to me, 'Bernard you really do believe, don't you, in "something over the rainbow?"'

'Yes, I do,' I said.

'Well, do you have any proof?'

'No. If you want a sign, you'll get it. But no proof.'

'Well,' said Charlie, 'when you return at Christmas, David asked that we scatter his ashes on the beach in Benidorm, where we all met.'

In December invited friends gathered at sunset on the beach and scattered David's ashes, as requested. There were about eight of us; others, not invited to be part of the service, stood about 50 yards back on the promenade, watching. They reported that, as we gathered, a lavender balloon was floating in the sky from the other end of the beach, unnoticed by us. During the 10 minute ritual it floated directly above our heads and remained there. At the end of the service, each one of us scattered a handful of David's ashes into the sea; whilst scattering the ashes, Charlie said, 'David, I'll always love you.' The lavender balloon landed at his feet.

A person becomes what they are open to. Belief in a higher power, or whatever we call it, is like belief in Santa Claus – he only comes when you believe in him! It could be fear, and dread of the void, that forces us to call it God! So what? Hope is, I believe, always better than despair. Clinical experience demonstrates people with a positive belief system have better mental and physical health than those without. As Viktor Frankl puts it in his inspiring account of his time in a Nazi concentration camp: 'Love does go very far beyond the physical person. It finds its deepest meaning in his spiritual being, his inner self' (Frankl 1969: 60).

The conflation of religion with spirituality and the failure of churches to embrace same sex sexuality instils a fear of anything connected to spirituality, thereby retarding the person's spiritual development. In extreme cases this causes a total rejection of their spirituality, a splitting or dissociation. The person can deny the spiritual part of their self (their soul, or psyche) becoming anti-spiritual, impoverishing themselves further in a context where they are already stigmatized.

The therapist must provide the client with the means to reflect on the socio-religious images of spirituality they have received and their actual experiences of the spiritual self. Together client and therapist can explore positive aspects, redefine negative ones and develop an affirming model of the spirit. This process can be extremely painful and involve the deconstruction of the client's 'god'. Very often this god has only been a disapproving or punitive force in their life. At the youngest age, many have been forced to choose between the integration of their self and sexuality and the god presented to them by church, family, culture. Put quite simply, either God goes or the person goes. This huge conflict creates a spiritual lacuna. The therapist working psychospiritually is engaged in guiding the client back to themselves.

Case example 3
Tom came to see me as a result of being diagnosed HIV positive in 1992. A married man with two daughters, with a very public position in the church in Scotland, Tom, like so many others, was initially in complete denial about his diagnosis. He wanted to deal immediately with issues of meaning: spirituality! My approach in such situations is simply to ask, 'What are you feeling right now? What is going on for you?' Tom quickly shared that his primary feeling was one of great fear.

During the third session, he started to talk about his sexual life, around which he had many feelings of guilt, not only in relation to his wife – with whom he was still living – but also to his current male partner. Both partners were aware of his diagnosis. Tom had concluded that his HIV positive status was a 'punishment' for his sexual and relational lifestyle. This is unsurprising in view of the homophobic pronouncements about HIV from Christian fundamentalists and certain sections of the media.

Tom had grown up in the northwest of Scotland in the late 1940s and early 1950s. Like so many of his generation he saw no alternative than to marry and settle down. From the beginnings of their courtship he had informed his wife of his gay sexuality. Arriving in Edinburgh in the 1970s, Tom engaged in a multiplicity of sexual encounters; often, he told me, 10 to 20 different partners a month. His sexual behaviour became obsessive and compulsive.

Three months into therapy he began to deal with his feelings of self-loathing which were compounded by his socio-religious culture. As a young boy he could 'never, ever please' either his father or his mother. He never felt he 'was the boy they tried to make [him] out to be'. Consequently he engaged surreptitiously in activities to 'get back at them by being naughty'. This pre-pubescent naughtiness had taken the form of him playing with his genitals. I asked him whether he fantasized when engaging in sexual activities. He told me that the first time he had fellatio as the active partner, he fantasized, particularly as he reached orgasm, getting back at his father, to the point of silently verbalizing 'Take this father! Take it! Take it! Take it! Fuck you, I am a man!' At this point in the session he broke down and cried at length. Later, Tom described this catharsis as one of the 'most profound experiences' of his life. Similar fantasies and verbalizations accompanied his activities into his late 20s.

Tom began to see that, at one level, his searching sexually was really about that approval, that acceptance he had not received from either parent and in particular, from his father. From that session on he was able to share his sexuality with much greater trust of my understanding and acceptance. He began gradually to accept and to value his child self, for whom for so long and so often he had sought approval and acceptance outside himself. Tom also became more realistic in terms of his prognosis and eventually, with his wife Nan, and his partner James, drew up his will and conveyed plans for his funeral service. He shared with his daughters his discovery of understanding the reasons for being so sexually active throughout his life and how he had learned to 'forgive' and accept himself within the discourse of his psychosexual history. His self-acceptance was a spiritual apotheosis, acknowledging his intrinsic goodness. Tom was accepting God in himself. He was now freed to engage with his own spiritual journeying towards peace with himself, which is the same as being at peace with God.

Tom stayed in therapy with me until he became too physically ill to see me. At that time, our sessions had moved further into the psychospiritual realm, where he talked through his questions about God, afterlife, meaning and so on. I visited him several times in the hospital before he died.

Discussion

I hope it will be obvious to the reader that my therapy relies heavily on a Rogerian non-judgemental, client-centred approach. At varying times, given the nature of the subject, I would be using frameworks offered by Jung (1933), May (1953), Erikson (1965), Fromm (1965) and Frankl (1969) in my therapeutic work with awareness.

Tom's insight into his obsessive–compulsive sexual behaviour awakened his recognition of self-betrayal as well as his disregard of the welfare of others. Any genuine relationship requires that the participants have self-knowledge and self-awareness, otherwise all contact with others becomes a pretence. By contrast, two people aware of themselves and of each other will increase self-awareness and personal identity through interaction. Stephanie Dowrick's *Intimacy and Solitude* (1991) is very good on the interrelationship between self-awareness and developing successful relations with others, as is Dorothy Rowe's work (see also Appendix 3).

From a Rogerian point of view, insight in psychotherapy is always defined by awareness of experience. Interpretation or explanation are rejected as inhibiting real growth. This way of perceiving was for Tom both the foundation and result of new learning with little to do with intellectual presentation. Rogers (1951) calls this the *primary technique*. Fundamental to the development of self-acceptance of attitudes, feelings and experiences, deep self-love is the ultimate reflection of insight. When insight refers not to theorizing but to the self-awareness implicit in conscious emotional experience, to direct contact with one's feeling towards another human being, then insight is very important for the therapeutic enterprise.

Over time, when Tom began to be in touch with his feelings of guilt and self-hatred and their connectedness to his need for fatherly loving, a breakthrough occurred, enabling him to reach out to his wife, his male partner and daughters in open communication. Within that process there were many episodes of silence expressive of the difficulties Tom experienced in this struggle. Silence, I believe, can be productive since emotional insight and grasp of experience often occur during prolonged periods of silence. The distinction between profound knowledge of oneself and insight into one's surroundings is artificial. We are examining questions of Being and our reason for being. This ontological discourse is not part of everyday language. Therapist and client struggle together to reveal what is happening spiritually. One reason, I believe, that music is universally accepted across class, culture and sexuality is that it is a language of the spirit rather than of reason. The therapist needs to conduct, to elicit the client's experiences and to reflect their mood and meaning. Ultimately the client determines the language which frees them to experience, to express and to be most truly themselves. Tom's realistic acceptance of his terminal condition and his movement into planning with, and for, others in relation to his approaching death were signs of the degree to which he had arrived in his journey. His insights in psychotherapy which led to self-acceptance became, in theological language, his acceptance of God and God's will for him in love eternal.

Conclusion

- The impact of organized religions has been unhelpful or destructive towards lesbian, gay and bisexual people and their spiritual development.
- Many people wish to separate such oppression from a search for meaning – their psychospiritual growth, their search for God in themselves.
- The conflation of religion with spirituality has led many clients to dissociate from their spiritual self and therapists can help deconstruct this dynamic and develop empowering and affirmative models of spirituality with the client to heal this impoverishment.
- Re-education and undoing indoctrination may be necessary and bibliotherapy can be a useful tool here, especially in countering the effects of 'Bible bingo'.
- The ontological discourse, though often unfamiliar, is a rich field in which self-awareness and insight can grow and freer communion with others be established.

- Offering a humanist alternative to those in conflict between their 'faith' (religion) and their own integrity (including their sexuality) is inadequate.
- No mainstream Christian churches yet validate the expression of same sex love; this denies the godliness and goodness of lesbian, gay and bisexual people.
- As the churches' rituals and ceremonies exclude them entirely, it is vital for people of diverse sexualities to create and participate in their own rites.
- The search for spiritual insight is closely related to the search for identity; such insight is of great significance in the psychotherapeutic endeavour.

APPENDIX I

Resources

Heterosexual questionnaire (Rochlin 1992: 203–4)

1 What do you think caused your heterosexuality?
2 When and how did you first decide you were a heterosexual?
3 Is it possible that your heterosexuality is just a phase you may grow out of?
4 Is it possible that your heterosexuality stems from a neurotic fear of members of the same sex?
5 Isn't it possible that all you need is a good gay lover?
6 If heterosexuality is normal, why are a disproportionate number of mental patients heterosexual?
7 To whom have you disclosed your heterosexuality? How did they react?
8 The great majority of child molesters are heterosexuals (95 per cent). Do you really consider it safe to expose your children to heterosexual teachers?
9 Heterosexuals are noted for assigning themselves and each other to narrowly restricted, stereotyped sex roles. Why do you cling to such an unhealthy form of role playing?
10 Why do heterosexuals place so much emphasis on sex?
11 There seem to be very few happy heterosexuals. Techniques have been developed that you might be able to use to change your sexual orientation. Have you considered aversion therapy to treat your sexual orientation?
12 Why are heterosexuals so promiscuous?
13 Why do you make a point of attributing heterosexuality to famous people? Is it to justify your own heterosexuality?
14 If you've never slept with a person of the same sex, how do you know you wouldn't prefer that?
15 Why do you insist on being so obvious and making a public spectacle of your heterosexuality? Can't you just be what you are and keep it quiet?

Association for Lesbian, Gay and Bisexual Psychologies leaflet

FINDING A GAY AFFIRMATIVE PSYCHOTHERAPIST OR COUNSELLOR

The Association for Lesbian, Gay and Bisexual Psychologies is the British section of a Europe wide organisation [ALGP Europe] of people professionally concerned to challenge homophobia and heterosexism in the field of psychology. This includes academic research, teaching and training, medical and psychiatric work and therapy and counselling practice. Our aims are printed on the back of this leaflet.

ALGBP-UK exists to promote equal opportunities and treatment for lesbian, gay and bisexual people within the field of psychology. This leaflet has been written for people seeking counselling or psychotherapy who identify, or feel they may want to identify, as gay, lesbian or bisexual, or who are presently questioning their sexuality and need support.

[Note: The terms 'Psychotherapist' or 'counsellor' are sometimes used interchangeably, so we have used the term 'practitioner' in this leaflet to mean both.]

What is a gay affirmative practitioner?

A therapist or counsellor who says they are gay affirmative is not saying they seek in any sense to encourage people to be homosexual or bisexual, but rather that they regard these sexualities as having *equal value with heterosexuality*. It is their role to help you express your sexuality, whatever it may be, in the ways you choose.

Why it is important to seek help from a gay affirmative practitioner?

ALGBP-UK believes that homosexual orientation should not be regarded as a problem or a sickness. We believe that it cannot be helpful for people who identify as homosexual or bisexual to seek help from any practitioner who believes these forms of sexual expression are unhealthy. If you seek help with a matter unconnected with your sexuality you should not be quizzed about your sexuality any more than a heterosexual person.

Many people feel uncertain at times over their sexuality, or it changes over time; in these instances, too, they will not be helped by someone who believes in a fixed sexuality or gives value to one form only.

Some may not view homosexuality or bisexuality as pathological [sick] but their experience of these things may be very limited. An ethical practitioner will let you know if they feel you need help they are not competent to give. They should also provide advice and suggestions as to where you might seek further help.

Should I seek a practitioner with a similar sexual orientation to my own?

Many lesbian, gay and bisexual people argue that it is not necessary to find a practitioner who is gay.

Many have found heterosexual practitioners who have been very able. Some prospective clients feel they would be more comfortable working with someone who has a similar sexuality. Clients have a right to ask about the practitioner's sexuality and therapists and counsellors should either disclose or explain why they choose not to. Whatever they say about their sexuality it is important that they are gay-affirmative and that you are able to trust and have a good rapport with the practitioner.

Where do I begin looking for a practitioner?

There are a number of registers of counsellors and therapists each with their own codes of ethics and entry requirements [eg BAC Directory, UKCP, BPS Directory of Chartered Psychologists]. There are also practitioners who are not registered.: this does not imply lack of competence. Your best policy is to ensure that you know what you want and to inform yourself of the available options before deciding who to see. These directories should be in reference libraries and the British Association for Counselling has a very useful helpline [01788 578328].

* Ask your GP what is available on the NHS.

* Contact your local social services department and ask what they have to offer.

* Your local Council for Voluntary Service or The Samaritans should be able to advise you on help in the voluntary sector.

* The independent sector mainly comprises individuals practising alone or within centres for alternative medicine. You may find lists of these on the registers mentioned above, Individual practitioners may be listed in Yellow Pages under 'Counselling', 'Psychotherapy' or 'Psychology'. They may advertise in the local or gay press. You may also get names through friends and acquaintances or through lesbian, gay or bisexual publications, helplines or other organisations.

* MIND produces an excellent leaflet called *Getting the best from your counsellor or psychotherapist*. Send a sae + 50p to MIND Publications, Granta House, 15-19 Broadway, London E15 4BQ

Some useful questions to ask

Please remember you need not ask *all* of these and the way *you* approach the practitioner will be important. Their answers are not nearly as important as the way in which they respond to you asking questions. Use your own judgement and notice how you feel with the person and their manner.

Initial telephone or person to person contact is vital for gathering information - for you and the practitioner. You need to know their fees and whether there is a sliding scale; when they could see you, for how long, with what commitment or timescale. What about cancelled appointments or rescheduling if you're ill? Ask about confidentiality and professional boundaries.

* How long have you been in practice?

* How would you describe your approach?

* What is your training? Was any of it about sexual orientation?

* Please tell me about your Code of Ethics.

* Do you have regular supervision and/or therapy?

* Have you worked on your own sexuality?

* What work have you done with lesbian, gay or bisexual clients before?

* How do you regard the lesbian or gay part of yourself?

NB We would not expect practitioners to answer all these questions but their approach to them will tell you a good deal. There are no right or wrong answers but by the end of the initial conversation you should have some idea of how caring, trustworthy and competent the person is.

After the first session...

You should leave the first session feeling that you have a sense of the practitioner as a person and as a competent professional. They should have listened to you and you should feel that they and you have some idea of how they can help you, what form that help will take and over approximately what period.

There are many theories and approaches in counselling and therapy so you should feel able to shop around and find one which suits you. No reputable practitioner will object to your making telephone enquiries. If you are seeking help in the independent sector you should expect to pay for the first session but this does not commit you to taking further sessions.

Everyone who seeks help feels apprehensive but if you feel that a particular practitioner is not someone you can trust, or if you feel that they are disrespectful or patronising, or that they value heterosexuality above other sexualities then look for help elsewhere.

ALGBP-UK have produced a list of some 'gay affirmative' practitioners. To obtain a copy send a sae to: **ALGBP - UK, PO Box 7534, London NW1 0ZA**

THE AIMS OF THE ALGBP - UK

ALGBP - UK aims to challenge heterosexist and homophobic theories, assumptions and practices within the field of psychology. The aim is to do this by:

1   Promoting lesbian, gay and bisexual mental health.

2   Developing lesbian, gay and bisexual psychologies.

3   Drawing specific attention to lesbians in the field of psychology.

4   Promoting international communications among gay, lesbian and bisexual educators, therapists and researchers.

5   Developing forums to support gay, lesbian and bisexual workers within psychology and related fields.

6   Enhancing the lesbian, gay and bisexual affirmative aspects of scientific research, educational activities and clinical practice.

7   Fighting explicit and implicit biphobia, homophobia, racism and sexism within psychology and related fields.

8   Providing support for lesbian, gay and bisexual people working in homophobic environments and those coming out.

9   Providing a platform for new research, ideas and directions.

APPENDIX 2

Community resources

Agencies and helplines

The following contacts are a very brief selection of agencies which may be useful for therapists or their clients. We have had to exercise a lot of restraint in selecting these few, and of course the current accuracy of these details was checked as we went to press. **Please check for yourself before giving the information to a client.**

Albert Kennedy Trust
23 New Mount Street
Manchester M4 4DE
0161 953 4059
Places young lesbians and gays who are homeless with selected and trained 'big brothers and sisters' (lesbian and gay foster parent project).

Association of Greater London Older Women (AGLOW)
formerly The Older Women's Project
The Manor Gardens Centre
6–9 Manor Gardens
London N7 6LA
Holds meetings for older lesbians at different accessible central London venues.

Association for Lesbian, Gay and Bisexual Psychologies (ALGBP)
P. O. Box 7534
London NW1 0ZA
Aims to support the development of gay affirmative psychology and provide training and referral to gay affirmative therapists. Has a referrals list of therapists outside London.

Bisexual Helpline
0181 569 7500 Tues and Weds 7.30–9.30 p.m.
0131 557 3620 Thurs 7.30–9.30 p.m.

Appendix 2

Black Lesbian and Gay Helpline
0171 620 3885 Tues–Thurs 2–4.30 p.m.

Deaf Lesbian and Gay Groups (DLAGGS)
c/o 7 Victoria Avenue
South Croydon
Surrey CR2 0QP
Minicom: 0181 660 2208 (evenings only)
A coordinating group to put deaf people in touch with their nearest lesbian, gay and bisexual support group.

Friends and Families of Lesbians and Gays (FFLAG)
P. O. Box 153
Manchester M60 1LP
A national network of telephone contacts who offer support to parents and partners of lesbians and gays.

Gay and Lesbian Legal Advice
Room N5, 10–14 Macklin Street
London WC2B 5NF
0171 831 3535 Mon–Fri 7–10 p.m.
Free legal advice by gay lawyers

Lesbian and Gay Bereavement Project
0181 455 8894
Telephone support for bereaved people. Possibility for face-to-face interviews in London.

Lesbian and Gay Christian Movement
Oxford House
Derbyshire Street
London E2 6HG
0171 739 1249
Counselling Helpline: 0171 739 8134 Wed and Sun 7–10 p.m.
Various caucuses and local groups.
There are also groups for Catholics, Jews, Quakers, Christian Scientists, Mormons, etc. See *Gay Times* for a full listing or call the Gay Switchboard.

Lesbian and Gay Foster and Adoptive Parents Network
c/o London Friend
86 Caledonian Road
London N1
Support group with information on adoption and fostering agencies.

Lesbian Information Service (LIS)
P. O. Box 8
Todmorden
Lancashire OL14 5TZ
01706 817235
LIS produces reading lists on a variety of topics: alcohol and women; young lesbians; education; etc.

London Lesbian and Gay Switchboard
0171 837 7324
24 hour telephone information and advice staffed by lesbian and gay volunteers.

National AIDS Helpline
0800 567123
24 hour free helpline for people concerned about HIV/AIDS.

National Friend
BM National Friend
London WC1N 3XX
Coordinating organization for local lesbian, gay and bisexual counselling and befriending services. See also under 'Friend' or 'Gay' in your local telephone directory.

Project for Advice, Counselling and Education (PACE)
34 Hartham Road
London N7 9JL
0171 700 1323
A London based counselling organization for lesbians and gay men. Provides crisis, short and long term individual and group therapy. Also an outreach service to people physically restricted by HIV/AIDS. Has a referrals list of therapists outside London.

Regard
c/o BM Regard
London WC1N 3XX
A national campaigning and support organization of lesbian, gay and bisexual disabled people.

There are also political and campaigning organizations; all political parties have a lesbian, gay and bisexual group. Most trade unions also have a lesbian, gay and bisexual group (Unison being the largest). A number of professions have lesbian and gay groups including medics, lawyers, teachers, etc.

There are currently lesbian and gay community centres in Edinburgh, Leicester, Manchester and a black lesbian and gay centre in London.

Non-gay specialist organizations referred to in chapters

Women's Health
52 Featherstone Street
London EC1Y 8RT
0171 251 6580

Human Fertilisation and Embryology Authority
Paxton House
30 Artillery Lane
London E1 7LS
0171 377 5077

Pregnancy Advisory Service (PAS)
11–13 Charlotte Street
London W1P 1HD
0171 637 8962

216 Appendix 2

Domestic Violence Intervention Project: Violence Prevention Programme
P. O. Box 2838
London W6 9ZE
0181 563 7983

Domestic Violence Intervention Project: Women's Support Service
P. O. Box 2838
London W6 9ZE
0181 748 6512

Institute for the Study of Drug Dependence (ISDD)
Waterbridge House
32–36 Loman Street
London SE1 OEE
0171 928 1211

Alcohol Concern
Waterbridge House
32–36 Loman Street
London SE1 0EE
0171 928 7377

Newspapers and magazines

Gay Times
Worldwide House
116–134 Bayham Street
London NW1 0BA
A monthly magazine aims to cover news and views from a national perspective. Available by subscription. Useful for up to date support agency listings. We would recommend it as a good way for heterosexual therapists to stay current with what is happening in the lesbian and gay communities.

The Pink Paper
77 City Garden Row
London N1 8EZ
A national free weekly newspaper available from gay venues and some alternative bookshops, libraries and community centres.

Diva
77 City Garden Row
London N1 8EZ
A monthly magazine for lesbians from the publishers of *The Pink Paper*

Gay Scotland
c/o 58a Broughton Street
Edinburgh EH1 3SA
A monthly magazine for lesbian, gay and bisexual people living and working in Scotland.

Bi Community News
BM Ribbit
London WC1N 3XX

APPENDIX 3

Books for clients and counsellors

We have divided this supplementary reading list into sections relating to the relevant chapters. Some books will be relevant to more than one chapter, and we have placed the books relating to the *fundamental issues* section together. References cited in the text will be found in the References section, following this Appendix.

All of the following are recommended reading for counsellors and therapists. Some of these books may be appropriate for clients as well. All of the books recommended for clients would be of use to therapists, and we suggest therapists only recommend a book after having read it first themselves.

This list has been compiled by the editors and contributors and by Paud Hegarty of Gay's the Word Bookshop from whom all these books are available. The bookshop can supply by mail order. Contact: Gay's the Word Bookshop, 66 Marchmont Street, London WC1N 1AB Tel: 0171 278 7654.

Fundamental issues

Babuscio, J. (1976) *We Speak for Ourselves – Experiences in Homosexual Counselling*. London: SPCK.
Blumenfeld, W. J. (ed.) (1992) *Homophobia: How We All Pay the Price*. Boston, MA: Beacon Press.
Boston Lesbian Psychologies Collective (ed.) (1987) *Lesbian Psychologies – Explorations and Challenges*. Urbana, IL: University of Illinois Press.
Burston, P. and Richardson, C. (eds) (1995) *A Queer Romance: Lesbians, Gay Men and Popular Culture*. London: Routledge.
Clark, D. (1987) *The New Loving Someone Gay*. Berkeley, CA: Celestial Arts.
Coleman, E. (ed.) (1988) *Integrated Identity for Gay Men and Lesbians: Psychotherapeutic Approaches for Emotional Well-Being*. New York: Harrington Park Press.
de Cecco, J. P. (ed.) (1984) *Bisexual and Homosexual Identities: Critical Clinical Issues*. New York: Haworth Press.

de Cecco, J. P. (ed.) (1988) *Gay Relationships.* New York: Harrington Park Press.
de Cecco, J. P. and Elia, J. P. (eds) (1993) *If You Seduce a Straight Person, Can You Make Them Gay?* New York: Harrington Park Press.
Duberman, M., Vicinus, M. and Chauncey, G. (1989) *Hidden from History: Reclaiming the Gay and Lesbian Past.* Harmondsworth: Penguin.
Dworkin, S. H. and Gutierrez, F. J. (eds) (1992) *Counseling Gay Men and Lesbians.* Alexandria, VA: American Counseling Association.
Falco, K. L. (1991) *Psychotherapy with Lesbian Clients: Theory into Practice.* New York: Brunner/Mazel.
Friedman, R. G. (1989) *Male Homosexuality: A Contemporary Psychoanalytic Perspective.* New Haven, CT: Yale University Press.
Geller, T. (ed.) (1990) *Bisexuality: A Reader and Sourcebook.* New York: Times Change Press.
Gever, M., Greyson, J. and Parmar, P. (1993) *Queer Looks: Perspectives on Lesbian and Gay Film and Video.* London: Routledge.
Gochros, J. (1989) *When Husbands Come Out of the Closet.* New York: Harrington Park Press.
Gonsiorek, J. C. (1989) *A Guide to Psychotherapy with Gay and Lesbian Clients.* New York: Harrington Park Press.
Gonsiorek, J. C. and Weinrich, J. D. (1991) *Homosexuality: Research Implications for Public Policy.* Newbury Park, CA: Sage Publications.
Greene, B. and Herek, G. M. (1994) *Lesbian and Gay Psychology: Theory, Research and Clinical Applications.* Newbury Park, CA: Sage Publications.
Greene, B. and Herek, G. M. (eds) (1996) *Ethnic and Cultural Diversity in the Lesbian and Gay Community.* Newbury Park, CA: Sage Publications.
Green, R. (1992) *The 'Sissy Boy' Syndrome and the Development of Homosexuality.* New Haven, CT: Yale University Press.
Hall, M. (1985) *The Lavender Couch: A Consumer's Guide to Psychotherapy for Lesbians and Gay Men.* Boston, MA: Alyson Publications.
Hall Carpenter Archives (1989) *Walking After Midnight: Gay Men's Life Stories.* London: Routledge.
Hall Carpenter Archives/Lesbian History Group (1989) *Inventing Ourselves: Lesbian Life Stories.* London: Routledge.
Hemphill, E. (1991) *Brother to Brother: New Writings by Black Gay Men.* Boston, MA: Alyson Publications.
Hutchins, L. and Kaahumanu (eds) (1991) *Bi Any Other Name: Bisexual People Speak Out.* Boston, MA: Alyson Publications.
Isay, R. A. (1989) *Being Homosexual – Gay Men and Their Development.* New York: Avon Books.
Klein, F. and Wolf, T. (1985) *Two Lives to Lead: Bisexuality in Men and Women.* New York: Harrington Park Press.
McKay, M. and Fanning, P. (1987) *Self-Esteem.* Oakland, CA: New Harbinger Publications.
Marcourt, M. (1989) *How Can We Help You: Information, Advice and Counselling for Gay Men and Lesbians.* London: Bedford Square Press.
Mason-John, V. (ed.) (1995) *Talking Black: Lesbians of African and Asian Descent Speak Out.* London: Cassell.
O'Connor, N. and Ryan, J. (1993) *Wild Desires and Mistaken Identities: Lesbianism and Psychoanalysis.* London: Virago.
Off Pink Collective (1988) *Bisexual Lives.* London: Off Pink Publishing.

Ross, M. W. (1988) *The Treatment of Homosexuals with Mental Health Disorders*. New York: Harrington Park Press.
Ross, M. W. (1989) *Psychopathology and Psychotherapy in Homosexuality*. New York: Haworth Press.
Shakespeare, T., Gillespie-Sells, K. and Davies, D. (1996) *The Sexual Politics of Disability: Untold Desires*. London: Cassell.
Silverstein, C. (1991) *Gays, Lesbians and Their Therapists: Studies in Psychotherapy*. New York: W. W. Norton.
Thompson, B. (1994) *Sadomasochism: Painful Perversion or Pleasurable Play?* London: Cassell.
Weinberg, G. (1972) *Society and the Healthy Homosexual*. New York: St Martin's Press.
Weinberg, W. (1994) *Dual Attraction*. Oxford: Oxford University Press.
Woodman, N. J. (ed.) (1992) *Lesbian and Gay Lifestyles – A Guide for Counselling and Education*. New York: Irvington Publishers.
Woodman, N. J. and Lenna, H. (1980) *Counselling with Gay Men and Women*. San Francisco, CA: Jossey Bass.
Young, V. (1995) *The Equality Complex: Lesbians in Therapy – a Guide to Anti-Oppressive Practice*. London: Cassell.

Specific issues

Chapter 4: Working with people coming out

Martin, E. (1993) *Is It a Choice?* New York: HarperCollins.
Penelope, J. and Valentine, S. (1990) *Finding the Lesbians: Personal Accounts from Around the World*. Freedom, CA: Crossing Press.
Signorile, M. (1995) *Outing Yourself*. New York: Random House.

Chapter 5: Working with single people

Berzon, B. (1990) *Permanent Partners – Building Gay and Lesbian Relationships That Last*. New York: Penguin Books (USA).
Driggs, J. H. and Finn, S. E. (1991) *Intimacy Between Men – How to Find and Keep Gay Love Relationships*. New York: Plume (Penguin Books).
Hart, J. (1991) *Gay Sex – A Manual for Men Who Love Men*. Boston, MA: Alyson Publications.
Isensee, R. (1991) *Growing Up Gay in a Dysfunctional Family*. Englewood Cliffs, NJ: Prentice Hall.
Loulan, J. A. (1984) *Lesbian Sex*. San Francisco, CA: Spinsters/Aunt Lute.
Rothblum, E. and Cole, E. (eds) (1989) *Loving Boldly: Issues Facing Lesbians*. New York: Harrington Park Press.
Tessina, T. (1989) *Gay Relationships: How to Find Them, How to Improve Them, How to Make Them Last*. Los Angeles, CA: Jeremy P. Tarcher Inc.

Chapter 6: Working with people in relationships

Burch, B. (1993) *On Intimate Terms*. Bloomington, IN: Indiana University Press.
Carl, D. (1990) *Counselling Same-Sex Couples*. New York: W. W. Norton.
Clunis, D. M. and Green, G. D. (1988) *Lesbian Couples*. Seattle, WA: Seal Press.

Isensee, R. (1990) *Love Between Men – Enhancing Intimacy and Keeping Your Relationship Alive.* Englewood Cliffs, NJ: Prentice Hall Press.
Marshall, A. (1995) *Together Forever? The Gay Guide to Good Relationships.* London: Pan.
Smith, R. K. and Tessina, T. B. (1987) *How to Be a Couple and Still Be Free.* North Hollywood, CA: Newcastle Publishing Co.

Chapter 7: Lesbian and gay parenting issues

Barrett, R. L. and Robinson, B. E. (1990) *Gay Fathers.* Lexington, KY: Lexington Books.
Martin, A. (1991) *The Lesbian and Gay Parenting Handbook.* London: Pandora Press.
Newman, L. (1991) *Heather Has Two Mommies.* Boston, MA: Alyson Publications.
Pies, C. (1988) *Considering Parenthood.* San Francisco, CA: Spinsters Book Company.
Pollack, S. (ed.) (1989) *Politics of the Heart.* Ithaca, NY: Firebrand.
Rights of Women Lesbian Custody Group (1992) *Lesbian Mothers' Legal Handbook.* London: The Women's Press.
Saffron, L. (1994) *Challenging Conceptions: Planning a Family by Self-Insemination.* London: Cassell.

Chapter 8: Working with young people

Epstein, D. (1994) *Challenging Lesbian and Gay Inequalities in Education.* Buckingham: Open University Press.
Grima, T. (ed.) (1994) *Not the Only One: Lesbian and Gay Fiction for Teens.* Boston, MA: Alyson Publications.
Harbeck, K. (ed.) (1993) *Coming Out of the Classroom Closet: Gay and Lesbian Students, Teachers and Curricula.* New York: Haworth Press.
Harris, S. (1990) *Lesbian and Gay Issues in the English Classroom.* Milton Keynes: Open University Press.
Lovell, A. (1995) *When Your Child Comes Out.* London: Sheldon Press.
McDonald, H. and Steinhorn, A. (1990) *Understanding Homosexuality – A Guide for Those Who Know, Love or Counsel Gay and Lesbian Individuals.* Oxford: Crossroad Publishing.
Sanderson, T. (1991) *A Stranger in the Family.* London: The Other Way Press.
Wardlaw, C. (1995) *One in Every Family: Dispelling the Myths About Lesbians and Gay Men.* Dublin: Basement Press.

Chapter 9: Working with older lesbians

Adelman, J. (1993) *Lamda Grey: A Practical, Emotional and Spiritual Guide for Gays and Lesbians Who Are Growing Older.* North Hollywood, CA: Newcastle Publishing Co.
Adelman, M. (1986) *Long Time Passing: Lives of Older Lesbians.* Boston, MA: Alyson Publications.
Kehoe, M. (1990) *Lesbians Over 60 Speak for Themselves.* New York: Haworth Press.
Neild, S. and Pearson, R. (1992) *Women Like Us.* London: Women's Press.

Chapter 10: Working with older gay men

Berger, R. M. (1982) *Gay and Gray: The Older Homosexual Gay Man*. Champaign, IL: University of Illinois Press.
Lee, J. A. (ed.) (1991) *Gay Midlife and Maturity*. New York: Harrington Park Press.

Chapter 11: Alcohol and substance misuse

Awiah, J. et al. (1992) *Race, Gender and Drug Services*, ISDD Research Monograph No. 6. London: ISDD.
Bennett, G. (ed.) (1989) *Treating Drug Users*. London: Routledge.
Institite for the Study of Drug Dependence (ISDD) (1983) *Drug Misuse Wall Chart*. London: ISDD.
Institute for the Study of Drug Dependence (ISDD) (1994) *Drug Abuse Briefing*. London: ISDD.
Institute for the Study of Drug Dependence (ISDD) (1994) *Shades of Grey*. London: ISDD (video package; running time 35 minutes. Includes *Drug Abuse Briefing* and a training booklet).
Tyler, A. (1988) *Street Drugs*. Sevenoaks: New English Library.

Chapter 12: Partner abuse

Burstow, B. (1992) *Feminist Therapy: Working in the Context of Violence*. Newbury Park, CA: Sage.
Island, D. and Letellier, P. (1991) *Men Who Beat the Men Who Love Them: Battered Men and Domestic Violence*. New York: Haworth.
Chandler, T. and Taylor, J. (1995) *Lesbians Talk: Violent Relationships*. London: Scarlet Press.

Chapter 13: Religious and spirituality conflicts

Glaser, C. (1990) *Come Home! Reclaiming Spirituality and Community as Gay Men and Lesbians*. New York: Harper and Row.
Goss, R. (1993) *Jesus Acted Up*. San Francisco: Harper.
Helminiak, D. A. (1994) *What the Bible Really Says About Homosexuality*. San Francisco, CA: Alamo Square Press.
McNeil, J. (1976) *The Church and the Homosexual*. Sheed, Andrews and McMell.
McNeil, J. (1988) *Taking a Chance on God: Liberating Theology for Gays, Lesbians and Their Lovers, Families and Friends*. Boston, MA: Beacon Press.
O'Neill, C. (1992) *Coming Out Within*. San Francisco: Harper.
Rowe, D. (1987) *Beyond Fear*. London: Fontana.
Rowe, D. (1988) *The Successful Self*. London: Fontana.
Rowe, D. (1991) *Wanting Everything: The Art of Happiness*. London: HarperCollins.
Stewart, E. (1992) *Daring to Speak Love's Name*. London: Hamish Hamilton.
Thompson, M. (ed.) (1995) *Gay Soul: Finding the Heart of Gay Spirit and Nature*. London: HarperCollins.

References

Alcorn, K. (1992) Queer and now. *Gay Times.* May: 20.
Allport, G. W. (1954) *The Nature of Prejudice.* Reading, MA: Addison-Wesley.
American Psychiatric Association (1980) *Diagnostic and Statistical Manual of Mental Disorders*, 3rd edn. Washington, DC. American Psychiatric Association. Revised 1987.
Amundson, J., Stewart, K. and Valentine, L. (1993) Temptations of power and certainty. *Journal of Family and Marital Therapy*, 19(2): 111–23.
Barnes, M. and Maple, N. (1992) *Women and Mental Health: Challenging the Stereotypes.* London: Venture.
Bass, E. and Davis, L. (1988) *The Courage to Heal: A Guide for Women Survivors.* London: Mandarin.
Beard, J. and Glickauf-Hughes, C. (1994) Gay identity and sense of self: rethinking male homosexuality. *Journal of Gay and Lesbian Psychotherapy*, 2(2): 21–37.
Beckett, E. (1989) Personal history, in Hall Carpenter Archives/Lesbian History Group (eds) *Inventing Ourselves.* London: Routledge.
Begelman, D. A. (1975) Ethical and legal issues of behavior modification, in M. Hersen, R. Eisler and P. M. Miller (eds) *Progress in Behavior Modification.* New York: Academic Press.
Beiber, I., Dain, H. J. and Dince, P. R. (1962) *Homosexuality: A Psychoanalytic Study of Male Homosexuals.* New York: Basic Books.
Bell, A. P. and Weinberg, M. S. (1978) *Homosexualities: A Study of Diversity Among Men and Women.* New York: Simon and Schuster.
Bennett, K. C. and Thompson, N. L. (1991) Accelerated ageing and male homosexuality, in J. A. Lee (ed.) *Gay Midlife and Maturity.* New York: Harrington Park Press.
Bernard, D. (1992) Developing a positive self-image in a homophobic environment, in N. J. Woodman (ed.) *Lesbian and Gay Lifestyles.* New York: Irvington Publishers Inc.
Bernstein, B. (1990) Attitudes and issues of parents of gay men and lesbians and implications for therapy. *Journal of Gay and Lesbian Psychotherapy*, 1(3): 37–53.

Berzon, B. (1990) *Permanent Partners: Building Lesbian and Gay Relationships That Last.* New York: Penguin Books.
Bion, W. (1965) *Transformations.* London: Heinemann.
Blair, R. (1982) *Ex-gay.* New York: Homosexual Counselling Center.
Bland, L. (1983) Purity, motherhood, pleasure or threat? definitions of female sexuality 1900–1970s, in C. Cartledge and J. Ryan (eds) *Sex and Love: New Thoughts on Old Contradictions.* London: Women's Press.
Bloomfield, K. (1993) A comparison of alcohol consumption between lesbians and heterosexual women in an urban population. *Drug and Alcohol Dependence,* 33: 257–69.
Blumenfeld, W. J. (1992) *Homophobia: How We All Pay The Price.* Boston: Beacon Press.
Blumenfeld, W. J. and Raymond, D. (1988) *Looking at Gay and Lesbian Life.* Boston: Beacon Press.
Blumstein, P. and Schwartz, P. (1983) American couples, in B. Green and G. M. Herek (eds) *Lesbian and Gay Psychology, Theory and Research Implications.* London: Sage.
Boden, R. (1992) Psychotherapy with physically disabled lesbians, in S. H. Dworkin and F. J. Gutierrez (eds) *Counseling Gay Men and Lesbians: Journey to the End of The Rainbow.* Alexandria, VA: American Counseling Association.
Boswell, J. (1980) *Christianity, Social Tolerance and Homosexuality: Gay People in Western Europe from the Beginning of the Christian Era to the Fourteenth Century.* Chicago: University of Chicago Press.
Boswell, J. (1989) Homosexuality and religious life: a historical approach, in J. Grammick (ed.) *Homosexuality in the Priesthood and the Religious Life.* New York: Crossroads.
Boswell, J. (1994) *Same Sex Unions in Premodern Europe.* New York: Villars Books.
Boxer, A. M. (1988) Betwixt and between: developmental discontinuities of gay and lesbian youth. Paper presented at the Society for Research on Adolescence, Alexandria, VA, March.
Brand, P. A., Rothblum, E. D. and Solomon, L. J. (1992) A comparison of lesbians, gay men and heterosexuals in weight and restrained eating, in B. Green and G. M. Herek (eds) *Lesbian and Gay Psychology, Theory and Research Implications.* London: Sage.
Bremner, J. and Hillin, A. (1993) *Sexuality, Young People and Care: Creating a Positive Context for Training, Policy and Development.* London: Central Council for Education and Training in Social Work (CCETSW), London and South East Region.
British Association for Counselling (BAC) (1992) *Code of Ethics and Practice for Counsellors,* amended September 1993. Rugby: BAC.
Buhrke, R. A. (1989) Incorporating lesbian and gay issues into counselor training: a resource guide. *Journal of Counseling and Development,* 68: 77–80.
Burbidge, M. and Walters, J. (eds) (1981) *Breaking the Silence: Lesbian and Gay Teenagers Speak Out.* London: Joint Council for Gay Teenagers.
Burch, B. (1982) Psychological merger in lesbian couples: a joint ego psychological and systems approach. *Family Therapy,* 9: 201–8.
Burgner, M. (1994) Working with the HIV patient: a psychoanalytic approach. *Psychoanalytic Psychotherapy,* 8: 201–13.
Burke, M. (1993) *Coming Out of the Blue: British Police Officers Talk About Their Lives in the Job as Lesbians, Gays and Bisexuals.* London: Cassell.

Burstow, B. (1992) *Feminist Therapy: Working in the Context of Violence*. Newbury Park, CA: Sage.
Burtle, V. (ed.) (1979) *Women Who Drink*. Springfield, IL: Charles C. Thomas.
Cameron, P. (1985) Homosexual molestation of children/sexual interaction of teacher and pupil. *Psychological Reports*, 57: 1227–36.
Cameron, P., Procter, K., Coburn, W., Jr., Forde, N., Larson, H. and Cameron, K. (1986) Child molestation and homosexuality. *Psychological Reports*, 58: 327–37.
Caprio, F. (1954) *Female Sexuality*. New York: Evergreen Black Cat.
Card, C. (ed.) (1992) *Hypatia* 7(4) Lesbian philosophy. Indiana University.
Carl, D. (1990) *Counseling Same-Sex Couples*. New York: Norton.
Cass, V. C. (1979) Homosexual identity formation: a theoretical model. *Journal of Homosexuality*, 4: 219–35.
Catalan, J. (1992) The psychosocial impact of HIV infection in gay men: a controlled investigation and factors associated with psychiatric morbidity. *British Journal of Psychiatry*, 161: 774–8.
Cayleff, S. (1986) Ethical issues in counselling gender, race and culturally distinct groups. *Journal of Counseling Development*, 64(5): 345–7.
Chodorow, N. (1994). *Feminism, Masculinities, Sexualities: Freud and Beyond*. London: Free Associations.
Chou, S. P. (1994) Sex differences in morbidity among respondents classified as alcohol users and/or dependent: results of a national survey. *Addiction*, 89: 87–93.
Churchill, W. (1967) *Homosexual Behaviour Among Males: A Cross-cultural and Cross-species Investigation*. New York: Hawthorn.
Clark, D. (1987) *The New Loving Someone Gay*. Berkeley, CA: Celestial Arts.
Clark, W. B. and Midanik, L. (1982) Alcohol use and alcohol problems among US adults: results of the 1979 national survey, in National Institute of Alcohol Abuse and Alcoholism (eds) *Alcohol and Health: Alcohol Consumption and Related Problems*. Washington DC: National Institute of Alcohol Abuse and Alcoholism.
Clunis, D. G. and Green, D. (1988) *Lesbian Couples*. Seattle, WA: Seal Press.
Cochrane, R. (1989) *Drinking Problems in Minority Ethnic Groups*. School of Psychology. University of Birmingham.
Cohen, C. and Stein, T. (1986) Reconceptualizing individual psychotherapy with gay men and lesbians, in C. Cohen and T. Stein, *Psychotherapy with Lesbians and Gay Men*. New York: Plenum Publishing Corp.
Cohen, E. (1991) Who are 'we'? Gay 'identity' as political (e)motion, in D. Fuss (ed.) *Inside/Out Lesbian Theories, Gay Theories*. New York: Routledge.
Coleman, E. (1981/82) Development stages of the coming out process. *Journal of Homosexuality*, 7: 31–43.
Coyle, A. (1993) A study of psychological well-being among gay men using the GHQ-30. *British Journal of Clinical Psychology*, 32: 218–20.
Coyle, A. (1994) Coming out sane: gay identity and mental health in adolescence. Paper presented to the National Children's Bureau Conference on Sexual Orientation in Adolescence. London 10 June.
Crain, W. C. (1985) *Theories of Development: Concepts and Applications*, 2nd edn. Englewood Cliffs, NJ: Prentice Hall.
Cramer, D. W. and Roach, A. J. (1988) Coming out to mom and dad: a study of gay males and their relationships with their parents. *Journal of Homosexuality*, 15(3/4): 79–91.

References 225

Cromwell, A. (1983) *Black Lesbians in White America*. Florida: Naiad Press.
Cronin, D. M. (1974) Coming out among lesbians, in E. Goode and R. Troiden (eds) *Sexual Deviance and Sexual Deviants*. New York: William Morrow.
D'Aguelli, A. R. (1989) Lesbian women in a rural helping network: exploring helping resources, in D. Rothblum and E. Cole (eds) *Lesbianism: Affirming Nontraditional Roles*. New York: Haworth Press.
Dank, B. M. (1973) 'The development of a homosexual identity: antecedents and consequences', unpublished doctoral dissertation, University of Wisconsin.
Davison, G. C. (1978) Not 'can' but 'ought'. The treatment of homosexuality. *Journal of Consulting and Clinical Psychology*, 46(1): 170–2.
Davison, G. C. (1991) Constructionism and morality in therapy for homosexuality, in J. C. Gonsiorek and J. D. Weinrich (eds) *Homosexuality: Research Implications for Public Policy*. Newbury Park, CA: Sage.
de Monteflores, C. (1986) Notes on the management of difference, in T. S. Stein and C. J. Cohen (eds) *Contemporary Perspectives on Psychotherapy with Lesbians and Gay Men*. New York: Plenum.
de Monteflores, C. and Schultz, S. J. (1978) Coming out. *Journal of Social Issues*, 34(3): 59–72.
Diamond, D. L. and Wilsnack, S. C. (1978) Alcohol abuse among lesbians: a descriptive study. *Journal of Homosexuality*, 4(2): 123–42.
Dollimore, J. (1991) *Sexual Dissidence*. Oxford: Clarendon.
Dörner, G. (1983) Letter to the editor. *Archives of Sexual Behaviour*, 12: 577–82.
Dowrick, S. (1991) *Intimacy and Solitude*. London: Women's Press.
Driggs, J. H. and Finn, S. E. (1991) *Intimacy Between Men – How to Find and Keep Gay Love Relationships*. New York: Plume/Penguin Books USA.
Duffy, M. (1967) *The Microcosm*. London: Panther.
Elfin Moses, A. (1990) Single lesbians and gays, in R. J. Kus (ed.) *Keys to Caring: Assisting Your Gay and Lesbian Clients*. Boston, MA: Alyson Publications.
Ellis, M. L. (1994) Lesbians, gay men and psychoanalytic training. *Free Associations*, 4(4): 501–17.
Epstein, D. (1994) *Challenging Lesbian and Gay Inequalities in Education*. Buckingham: Open University Press.
Erikson, E. (1946) Ego development and historical change. *The Psychoanalytic Study of the Child*, 2: 359–96.
Erikson, E. (1965) *Childhood and Society*. New York: International Universities Press.
Ernst, S. and Goodison, L. (1981) *In Our Own Hands: A Book of Self-Help Therapy*. London: Women's Press.
Espin, O. M. (1987) Issues of identity in the psychology of latina lesbians, in Boston Psychologies Collective (eds) *Lesbian Psychologies: Explorations and Challenges*. Urbana, IL: University of Illinois Press.
Etnyre, W. S. (1990) Body image and gay American men, in R. Kus (ed.) *Keys to Caring*. Boston, MA: Alyson Publications.
Fairlie, J., Nelson, J. and Popplestone, R. (1987) *Menopause – A Time for Positive Change*. London: Javelin.
Falco, K. L. (1991) *Psychotherapy with Lesbian Clients: Theory into Practice*. New York: Brunner/Mazel.
Farley, N. (1992) Same sex domestic violence, in S. H. Dworkin and F. J. Gutierrez (eds) *Counseling Gay Men and Lesbians: Journey to the End of the Rainbow*. Alexandria, VA: American Counseling Association.
Fay, R. E., Turner, C. F., Klassen, A. D. and Gagnon, J. H. (1989) Prevalence and patterns of same-gender sexual contact among men. *Science*, 243: 338–48.

Fifield, L. (1975) *On My Way to Nowhere: Alienated, Isolated, Drunk.* Los Angeles, CA: Gay Community Services Center.
Fine, M. and Asch, A. (1985) Disabled women: sexism without the pedestal, in B. Green and G. M. Herek (eds) *Lesbian and Gay Psychology, Theory and Research Implications.* London: Sage.
Forstein, M. (1988) Homophobia: an overview, *Psychiatric Annals,* 18(1): 33–6.
Foucault, M. (1981) Friendship as lifestyle: an interview, *Gay Information,* 7(4) spring.
Fox, M. (ed.) (1993) *Meditations with Meister Eckhart.* Santa Fe, NM: Bear and Co.
Frank, J. (1963) *Persuasion and Healing: A Comparative Study of Psychotherapy.* New York: Shocken Books.
Frankl, E. V. (1969) *The Will to Meaning.* New York: World Publishing.
Freud, S. (1905/1974) Three essays on the theory of sexuality, in A. Richards (ed.) *On Sexuality,* vol. VII of the Pelican Freud Library. Harmondsworth: Penguin.
Freud, S. (1913/1955) The claims of psycho-analysis to scientific interest, in J. Strachey (ed.) *The Standard Edition of Freud's Complete Psychological Works,* vol. 13. London: Hogarth Press.
Freud, S. (1947) Letter to an American mother. *American Journal of Psychiatry,* 107(51): 786–7.
Freund, K., Langevin, R., Gibiri, S. and Zajac, Y. (1973) Heterosexual aversion in homosexual males. *British Journal of Psychiatry.* 122: 163–9.
Freund, K. W. (1974) Male homosexuality: an analysis of the pattern, in J. A. Loraine (ed.) *Understanding Homosexuality: Its Biological and Psychological Bases.* New York: Elsevier: 25–81.
Friedman, R. C. (1988) *Male Homosexuality: A Contemporary Psychoanalytic Perspective.* New Haven, CT: Yale University Press.
Fromm, E. (1965) *Escape from Freedom.* New York: Avon Library.
Gebhard, P. H. (1972) Incidence of overt homosexuality in the United States and Western Europe, in J. J. Livingood (ed.) *NIMH Task Force on Homosexuality: Final Report and Background Papers.* DHEW publication no. (HSM) 72-9116. Rockville, MD: National Institute of Mental Health.
Gilroy, B. (1994) Black old age . . . the diaspora of the senses? in M. Wilson (ed.) *Health and Wise: The Essential Health Handbook for Black Women.* London: Virago.
Golombok, S., Spencer, A. and Rutter, M. (1983) Children in lesbian and single parent households: psychosexual and psychiatric appraisal. *Journal of Child Psychology Psychiatry,* 24: 551–72.
Gonsiorek, J. C. (1977) Psychological adjustment and homosexuality. *Social and Behavioural Science Documents,* MS 1478. San Raphael, CA: Select Press.
Gonsiorek, J. C. (1981) Review of homosexuality in perspective. *Journal of Homosexuality,* 6(3): 81–8.
Gonsiorek, J. C. (1988) Mental health issues of gay and lesbian adolescents. *Journal of Adolescent Health Care,* 9(2): 114–27.
Gonsiorek, J. C. and Rudolph, J. R. (1991) Homosexual identity: coming out and other development events, in J. C. Gonsiorek and J. D. Weinrich (eds) *Homosexuality: Research Implications for Public Policy.* Newbury Park, CA: Sage Publications.
Gonsiorek, J. C. and Weinrich, J. D. (1991) The definition and scope of sexual orientation, in J. C. Gonsiorek and J. D. Weinrich (eds) *Homosexuality: Research Implications for Public Policy.* Newbury Park, CA: Sage Publications.

Goode, E. and Haber, L. (1977) Sexual correlates of homosexual experience: an exploratory study of college women. *Journal of Sex Research*, 13: 12–21.

Grace, J. (1977) Gay despair and the loss of adolescence: a new perspective on same sex preference and self-esteem. Paper presented at the Fifth Biennial Professional Symposium of the National Association of Social Workers, San Diego, November.

Gramick, J. (1983) Homophobia: a new challenge. *Social Work*, 28(2): 137–41.

Grau, G. (1995) *The Hidden Holocaust: Gay and Lesbian Persecution in Germany, 1933–45*. London: Cassell.

Greasley, P. (1986) *Gay Men at Work*. London: Lesbian and Gay Employment Rights.

Green, R., Mandel, J. B., Horvedt, M. E., Gray, J. and Smith, L. (1986) Lesbian mothers and their children: a comparison with solo parent heterosexual mothers and their children. *Archives of Sexual Behaviour*, 15: 167–84.

Greene, B. and Herek, G. M. (eds) (1994) *Lesbian and Gay Psychology – Theory, Research and Clinical Applications*. Newbury Park, CA: Sage.

Groves, P. A. and Ventura, L. A. (1983) The lesbian coming out process: therapeutic considerations. *Personnel and Guidance Journal*, November: 146–9.

Gutierrez, F. J. (1992) Eros, the ageing years: counseling older gay men, in S. H. Dworkin and F. J. Gutierrez (eds) *Counseling Gay Men and Lesbians: Journey to the End of the Rainbow*. Alexandria, VA: American Counseling Association.

Haldeman, D. C. (1991) Sexual orientation conversion therapy for gay men and lesbians: a scientific examination, in J. C. Gonsiorek and J. D. Weinrich (eds) *Homosexuality: Research Implications for Public Policy*. Newbury Park, CA: Sage Publications.

Hall, M. (1985) *The Lavender Couch*. Boston, MA: Alyson Publications.

Hall, M. (1987) Reflections on the new lesbian (un)couple. Paper originally presented at a conference entitled 'Homosexuality – Which Homosexuality?' Amsterdam Free University, Amsterdam.

Hall, M. (1990) Lesbians and sex. Public address to Lesbians and Psychology Group, A Woman's Place, Wesley House, London.

Hall, R. (1928) *The Well of Loneliness*. London: Jonathan Cape.

Hall Carpenter Archives (1989) *Walking After Midnight: Gay Men's Life Stories*. London: Routledge.

Hall Carpenter Archives/Lesbian History Group (1989) *Inventing Ourselves: Lesbian Life Stories*. London: Routledge.

Hammond, N. (1989) Lesbian victims of relationship violence, in E. Rothblum and E. Cole (eds) *Loving Boldly: Issues Facing Lesbians*. New York: Harrington Park Press.

Hanley-Hackenbruck, P. (1989) Psychotherapy and the 'coming out' process. *Journal of Gay and Lesbian Psychotherapy*, 1(1): 21–39.

Harris, S. (1990) *Lesbian and Gay Issues in the English Classroom*. Milton Keynes: Open University Press.

Hart, M., Robrack, H., Tittler, B., Weitz, L., Walston, B., McKee, E. (1978) Psychological adjustment of nonpatient homosexuals: critical review of the research literature. *Journal of Clinical Psychiatry*, 39: 604–8.

Heather, N. and Robertson, I. (1989) *Problem Drinking: The New Approach*, 2nd edn. Oxford: Oxford Medical Publication.

Hedblom, J. H. (1973) Dimensions of lesbian sexual experience. *Archives of Sexual Behaviour*, 2: 329–41.

Helfand, K. L. (1993) Therapeutic considerations in structuring a support group

for the mentally ill gay/lesbian population. *Journal of Gay and Lesbian Psychotherapy*, 2(1): 65–76.
Hemmings, D. (1989) *Older Lesbians*, information leaflet. London: Lesbian Line.
Henker, F. O. (1979) Body image conflict following trauma and surgery, in R. Kus (ed.) *Keys To Caring*. Boston, MA: Alyson Publications.
Hepburn, G. and Gutierrez, B. (1988) *Alive and Well: A Lesbian Health Guide*. Freedom, CA: Crossing Press.
Herek, G. M. (1984) Beyond 'homophobia': a social psychological perspective on attitudes toward lesbians and gay men. *Journal of Homosexuality*, 10(1/2): 53–67.
Herek, G. M. (1991) Stigma, prejudice and violence against lesbians and gay men, in J. C. Gonsiorek and J. D. Weinrich (eds) *Homosexuality: Research Implications for Public Policy*. Newbury Park, CA: Sage Publications.
Hetrick, E. S. and Martin, A. D. (1987) Developmental issues and their resolution for gay and lesbian adolescents. *Journal of Homosexuality*, 14(1/2): 25–43.
Hildebrand, H. P. (1992) A patient dying with AIDS. *International Review of Psycho-Analysis*, 19: 457–69.
Hocquenghem, G. (1978) *Homosexual Desire*. London: Allison and Busby.
Holtzen, D. W. and Agresti, A. A. (1990) Parental responses to gay and lesbian children: difficulties in homophobia, self-esteem and sex-role stereotyping. *Journal of Social and Clinical Psychology*, 9(3): 390–9.
Hooker, E. A. (1957) The adjustment of the male overt homosexual. *Journal of Projective Techniques*, 21: 17–31.
Hudson, W. W. and Ricketts, W. A. (1980) A strategy for the measurement of homophobia. *Journal of Homosexuality*, 5(4): 317–72.
Iasenza, S. (1989) Some challenges of integrating sexual orientations into counselor training and research. *Journal of Counseling and Development*, 68: 73–6.
International Statistical Classification of Diseases and Related Health Problems (ICD) (1992) Tenth Revision. Geneva: World Health Organization.
Isay, R. A. (1986) On the analytic therapy of gay men, in T. S. Stein and C. J. Cohen (eds) *Contemporary Perspectives on Psychotherapy with Lesbians and Gay Men*. New York: Plenum Publishing.
Isay, R. A. (1989) *Being Homosexual: Gay Men and Their Development*. New York: Avon Books.
Isensee, R. (1990) *Love Between Men – Enhancing Intimacy and Keeping Your Relationship Alive*. Englewood Cliffs, NJ: Prentice Hall Press.
Jay, K. and Young, A. (1979) *The Gay Report: Lesbians and Gay Men Speak Out About Sexual Experiences and Lifestyles*. New York: Simon and Schuster.
Jeffreys, S. (1994) *The Lesbian Heresy: A Feminist Perspective on the Lesbian Sexual Revolution*. London: Women's Press.
Jourard, S. (1971) *The transparent self*. New York: D. Van Nostand.
Jung, C. J. (1933) *Modern Man in Search of a Soul*. New York: Harcourt, Brace and World.
Kimmel, D. C. (1978) Adult development and ageing: a gay perspective. *Journal of Social Issues*, 34(3): 113–30.
Kinsey, A. C., Pomeroy, W. B. and Martin, C. E. (1947) *Sexual Behavior in the Human Male*. Philadelphia, PA: W. B. Saunders.
Kinsey, A. C., Pomeroy, W. B., Martin, C. E. and Gebhard, P. H. (1953) *Sexual Behavior in the Human Female*. Philadelphia, PA: W. B. Saunders.
Kippax, S., Crawford, J., Connell, B., Dowsett, G., Watson, L., Rodden, P., Baxter, D. and Berg, R. (1992) The importance of gay community in the prevention

of HIV transmission: a study of Australian men who have sex with men, in P. Aggleton et al. (eds) *AIDS: Rights, Risks and Reason*. London: Falmer.

Kirsch, J. A. W. and Weinrich, J. D. (1991) Homosexuality, nature and biology: is homosexuality natural? does it matter? in J. C. Gonsiorek and J. D. Weinrich (eds) *Homosexuality: Research Implications for Public Policy*. Newbury Park, CA: Sage.

Kitzinger, C. (1989) Liberal humanism as an ideology of control: the regulation of lesbian identities, in J. Shotter and K. Gergen (eds) *Texts of Identity*. London: Sage.

Kitzinger, C. and Perkins, R. (1993) *Changing Our Minds: Lesbianism Feminism and Psychology*. London: OnlyWomen.

Klaich, D. (1974) *Woman Plus Woman: Attitudes Towards Lesbianism*. New York: Simon and Schuster.

Klein, C. (1991) *Counselling Our Own: The Lesbian/Gay Subculture Meets the Mental Health Service*, 2nd edn. Seattle: Consultant Services North West.

Krajeski, J. P. (1986) Psychotherapy with gay men and lesbians: a history of controversy, in T. S. Stein and C. J. Cohen (eds) *Contemporary Perspectives on Psychotherapy with Lesbians and Gay Men*. New York: Plenum.

Kübler-Ross, E. (1986) *On Death and Dying*. New York: Macmillan.

Kus, R. J. (1989) Bibliotherapy and the gay American men of Alcoholics Anonymous. *Journal of Lesbian and Gay Psychotherapy*, 1(2): 74.

Lago, C. and Thompson, J. (1989) Counselling and race, in W. Dryden, D. Charles Edwards and R. Woolfe. *Handbook of Counselling In Britain*. London: Routledge.

Langevin, R., Stanford, A. and Block, R. (1975) The effects of relaxation instructions on erotic arousal in homosexual and heterosexual males. *Behaviour Therapy*, 6: 3–58.

Le Vay, S. (1994) *The Sexual Brain*. London: A Bradford Book.

Lee, J. A. (ed.) (1991) *Gay Midlife and Maturity*. New York: Harrington Park Press.

Lehne, G. K. (1976) Homophobia among men, in D. S. David and R. Brannon (eds) *The Forty-nine Percent Majority: The Male Sex Role*. Reading, MA: Addison-Wesley.

Lendrum, S. and Syme, G. (1994) *Gift of Tears: A Practical Approach to Loss and Bereavement Counselling*. London: Routledge.

Levitt, E. E. and Klassen, A. D. (1974) Public attitudes toward homosexuality: Part of the 1970 national survey by the Institute of Sex Research. *Journal of Homosexuality*, 1(1): 29–43.

Lewes, K. (1988) *The Psychoanalytic Theory of Male Homosexuality*. New York: Simon and Schuster.

Lewis, R. A. (1978) Emotional intimacy among men. *Journal of Social Issues*, 34(1): 108–21.

Limentani, A. (1994) On the treatment of homosexuality, *Psychoanalytic Psychotherapy*, 8: 49–62.

Lindenfield, G. (1993) *Managing Anger: Positive Strategies in Dealing with Destructive Emotions*. Wellingborough: Thorsons.

Lohrenz, L., Connelly, J., Coyne, L., Spare, K. (1978) Alcohol problems in several midwestern homosexual communities. *Journal of Studies on Alcohol*, 39(11): 1959–63.

Loulan, J. (1991) 'Now when I was your age': one perspective on how lesbian culture has influenced our sexuality, in B. Sang, J. Warshow and A. J. Smith (eds) *Lesbians at Midlife: The Creative Transition.* San Francisco, CA: Spinsters Book Company.

Lynch, Dr B. (1993) *Priest on Trial.* London: Bloomsbury.

McDonald, G. J. (1982) Individual differences in the coming out process of gay men: implications for theoretical models. *Journal of Homosexuality*, 8(1): 47–60.

MacDonald, B. and Rich, C. (1985) *Look Me in the Eye: Old Women, Age and Ageism.* London: Women's Press.

McKirnan, D. J. and Peterson, P. L. (1988) Stress, expectations and vulnerability to substance use: a test of a model among homosexual men. *Journal of Abnormal Psychology*, 97(4): 461–6.

McKirnan, D. J. and Peterson, P. L. (1989) Alcohol and drug use among homosexual men and women: epidemiology and population characteristics. *Addictive Behaviors*, 14: 545–53.

McLellan, B. (1995) *Beyond Psychoppression.* Melbourne: Sphinx.

Manosevitz, M. (1970) Early sexual behaviour in adult homosexual and heterosexual males. *Journal of Abnormal Psychology*, 76: 396–402.

Margolies, L., Becker, M. and Jackson-Brewer, K. (1987) Internalized homophobia: identifying and treating the oppressor within, in Boston Lesbian Psychologies Collective (eds) *Lesbian Psychologies – Explorations and Challenges.* Chicago, IL: University of Illinois Press.

Marie (1992) Personal history, in S. Neild and J. Pearson, *Women Like Us.* London: Women's Press.

Martin, A. D. and Hetrick, E. S. (1988) The stigmatization of the gay and lesbian adolescent, in M. W. Ross (ed.) *The Treatment of Homosexuals with Mental Health Disorders.* New York: Harrington Park Press.

Mason-John, V. (ed.) (1995) *Talking Black: Lesbians of African and Asian Descent Speak Out.* London: Cassell.

Mason-John, V. and Khambatta, A. (1993) *Lesbians Talk: Making Black Waves.* London: Scarlett.

Masson, J. (1984) *The Assault on Truth.* New York: Farrar, Strauss and Giroux.

May, R. (1953) *Man's Search for Himself.* New York: Dell Publishing Co.

Maylon, A. (1982) Psychotherapeutic implications of internalized homophobia in gay men, in J. Gonsiorek (ed.) *Homosexuality and Psychotherapy.* New York: Haworth Press.

Mays, V. M., Cochran, S. D. and Rhue, S. (1993) The perceived discrimination on the intimate relationships of black lesbians. *Journal of Homosexuality*, 25(4): 1–14.

Mencher, J. (1990) *Intimacy in Lesbian Relationships: A Critical Re-Examination of Fusion.* Stone Center, Wellesley College, Wellesley, MA.

Messing, A. E., Schoenberg, R. and Stephens, R. K. (1984) Confronting homophobia in health care settings: guidelines for social work practice, in R. Schoenberg, R. S. Goldberg and D. A. Shore (eds) *Homosexuality and Social Work.* New York: Haworth Press.

Meyer, J. K. (1985) Ego-dystonic homosexuality, in H. Kaplan and B. Sadock (eds) *Comprehensive Textbook of Psychiatry IV.* Baltimore, MD: Williams and Wilkins.

Minton, H. and McDonald, G. J. (1983/84) Homosexual identity formation as a development process. *Journal of Homosexuality*, 9(2/3): 91–104.

Money, J. and Ehrhardt, A. A. (1972) *Man and Woman, Boy and Girl: Differentiation and Dimorphism of Gender Identity from Conception to Maturity.* Baltimore, MD: Johns Hopkins Press.

Morrow, S. L. and Hawxhurst, D. M. (1989) Lesbian partner abuse. Implications for therapists. *Journal of Counselling and Development*, 68: 58–62.
Moses, A. and Hawkins, R. (1982) *Counseling Lesbian Women and Gay Men: A Life-Issues Approach*. St Louis, MO: Mosby.
Mosher, D. L. (1991) Scared straight: homosexual threat in heterosexual therapists, in C. Silverstein (ed.) *Gays, Lesbians and their Therapists*. New York: W. W. Norton & Co.
Nardi, P. M. (1982) Alcoholism and homosexuality: a theoretical perspective. *Journal of Homosexuality*, 7(4): 9–25.
Neild, S. and Pearson, R. (1992) *Women Like Us*. London: Women's Press.
Neisen, J. H. (1990). Redefining homophobia for the 1990s. *Journal of Gay and Lesbian Psychotherapy*, 1(3): 21–35.
O'Connor, N. and Ryan, J. (1993) *Wild Desires and Mistaken Identities: Lesbianism and Psychoanalysis*. London: Virago Press.
Orbach, S. (1995) Beware the prejudiced analyst. *The Guardian: Weekend*, 29 April: 8.
Parmar, P. (1989) Black lesbians loving women: lesbian life and relationships, in A. Phillips *The New Our Bodies, Ourselves*. London: Penguin.
Pearce, W. B. (1989) *Communication and the Human Condition*. Edwardsville, IL: Southern Illinois University Press.
Phillips, A. and Rakusen, J. (eds) (1989) *Ourselves Growing Older*. London: Penguin.
Plummer, K. (1975) *Sexual Stigma: An Interactionist Account*. London: Routledge & Kegan Paul.
Prochaska, J. O. and Di Clemente, C. C. (1983) Transtheoretical therapy: towards a more integrative model of change. *Psychotherapy: Theory, Research and Practice*, 19: 276–88.
Rabin, J., Keefe, K. and Burton, M. (1986) Enhancing services to sexual minority clients: a community mental health approach. *Social Work*, 31(4): 294–8.
Ramsey, G. V. (1973) The sexual development of boys. *American Journal of Psychiatry*, 56: 217–34.
Raphael, B. (1984) *The Anatomy of Bereavement: A Handbook for the Caring Professions*. London: Hutchinson.
Ratigan, B. (1991) Personal communication.
Ratzinger, J. (1986) On pastoral care of homosexual people. Congregation for the Doctrine of the Faith, Vatican City, on Halloween, 31 October.
Reiss, B. F. (1980) Psychological tests in homosexuality, in J. Marmor (ed.) *Homosexual Behavior: A Modern Reappraisal*. New York: Basic Books.
Rivers, I. (1994) Protecting the gay adolescent in school. Paper at the 2nd International Congress on Adolescentology, Milan, 18–19 November.
Rivers, I. (1995a) The victimisation of gay teenagers in school: homophobia in education. *Pastoral Care in Education*, 13(1): 39–45.
Rivers, I. (1995b) Mental health issues among lesbians and gay men bullied in school. *Health and Social Care in the Community*, 3(6): 380–3.
Roberts, J. and Pines, M. (eds) (1991) *The Practice of Group Analysis*. London: Routledge.
Robinson, G. (1984) Few solutions for a young dilemma. *The Advocate*, pp. 14–16.
Rochlin, M. (1992) Heterosexual questionnaire, in W. J. Blumenfeld (ed.) *Homophobia: How We All Pay the Price*. Boston, MA: Beacon Press.
Rogers, C. (1951) *Client Centred Therapy*. Boston, MA: Houghton Mifflin.
Ross, M. W. (ed.) (1988) *The Treatment of Homosexuals with Mental Health Disorders*. New York: Harrington Park Press.

Ross-Reynolds, G. (1982) Issues of counseling the 'homosexual' adolescent, in J. Grimes (ed.) *Psychological Approaches to Problems of Children and Adolescents*. Des Moines, IA: Iowa State Department of Education.
Rothblum, E. D. (1990) Depression among lesbians: an invisible and unresearched phenomenon. *Journal of Lesbian and Gay Psychotherapy*, 1: 67–87.
Rothblum, E. D. and Cole, E. (eds) (1989) *Loving Boldly: Issues Facing Lesbians*. New York: Harrington Park Press.
Ruse, M. (1988) *Homosexuality*. Oxford: Blackwell.
Russell, J. (1993) *Out of Bounds*. Newbury Park, CA: Sage.
Russo, V. (1991) *The Celluloid Closet: Homosexuality in the Movies*. New York: Borgo Press.
Ruszczynski, S. (ed.) (1993) *Psychotherapy with Couples*. London: Karnac Books.
Rutter, P. (1990) *Sex in the Forbidden Zone*. London: Mandala/HarperCollins.
Ryan, J. (1983) Psychoanalysis and women loving women, in C. Cartledge and J. Ryan (eds) *Sex and Love: New Thoughts on Old Contradictions*. London: Women's Press.
Saghir, M. T. and Robins, E. (1973) *Male and Female Homosexuality: A Comprehensive Investigation*. Baltimore, MD: Williams and Wilkins Co.
Saghir, M. T., Robins, E., Walbran, B. and Gentry, K. A. (1970) Homosexuality IV: disorders and disability in the female homosexual. *American Journal of Psychiatry* 127(2): 147–54.
Sanderson, T. (1990) *Making Gay Relationships Work: A Handbook for Male Couples*. London: The Other Way Press.
Sanderson, T. (1993) *Assertively Gay: How to Build Gay Self-esteem*. London: The Other Way Press.
Sandmaier, M. (1980) *The Invisible Alcoholics: Women and Alcohol Abuse in America*. New York: McGraw-Hill.
Sang, B., Warshow, J. and Smith, A. J. (1991) *Lesbians at Midlife: The Creative Transition*. San Francisco, CA: Spinster's Book Company.
Savin-Williams, R. C. (1990) *Gay and Lesbian Youth: Expressions of Identity*. New York: Hemisphere Publishing Corporation.
Secord, P. F. and Backman, C. W. (1961) Personality theory and the problem of stability and change in individual behaviour: an interpersonal approach. *Psychological Review*, 68: 21–32.
Secord, P. F. and Backman, C. W. (1964) Effects of imbalance in the self-concept on the perceptions of persons. *Journal of Abnormal and Social Psychology*, 68: 442–6.
Secord, P. F. and Backman, C. W. (1974) *Social Psychology*, 2nd edn. Tokyo: McGraw-Hill Kogakusha.
Sell, R. L., Wells, J. A., Valleron, A-J., Will, A., Cohen, M. and Umbel, K. (1990) Homosexual and bisexual behavior in the United States, the United Kingdom and France. Paper presented at the Sixth International Conference on AIDS, San Francisco, CA, June.
Sergios, P. and Cody, J. (1985/86) Importance of physical attractiveness and assertiveness skills in male homosexual dating behavior and partner selection, in J. de Cecco *Gay Relationships*. New York: Harrington Park Press.
Shakespeare, T., Gillespie-Sells, K. and Davies, D. (eds) (1996) *The Sexual Politics of Disability: Untold Desires*. London: Cassell.
Shapiro, J. (1989) The menopause: entering our third age, in P. B. Doress and D. L. Siegal (eds) *Ourselves Growing Older*. London: Fontana.

Shepherd, S. and Wallis, M. (eds) (1989) *Coming on Strong: Gay Politics and Culture*. London: Unwin Hyman.
Shernoff, M. (1989) AIDS prevention counseling in clinical practice, in J. W. Dilley, C. Pies and M. Helquist (eds) *Face to Face: A Guide to AIDS Counseling*. University of California, AIDS Health Project.
Shields, S. A. and Harriman, R. E. (1984) Fear of male homosexuality: cardiac responses of low and high homonegative males. *Journal of Homosexuality*, 10(1/2): 53–67.
Shively, M. D., Jones, C. and De Cecco, J. P. (1983/84). Research on sexual orientation: definitions and methods. *Journal of Homosexuality*, 9(2/3): 127–36.
Signorile, M. (1994) *Queer in America: Sex, the Media and the Closets of Power*. New York: Anchor.
Silberstein, L., Mishkind, M., Striegal-Moore, R. and Timko, C. (1989) Men and their bodies: a comparison of homosexual and heterosexual men. *Psychosomatic Medicine*, 51: 337–46.
Silverstein, C. (1977) Homosexuality and the ethics of behavioural interventions: paper 2. *Journal of Homosexuality*, 2(3): 205–11.
Silverstein, C. (1988) The borderline personality disorder and gay people, *Journal of Homosexuality*, 15(1–2): 185–212.
Silverstein, C. (1991) Psychological and medical treatments of homosexuality, in J. C. Gonsiorek and J. D. Weinrich (eds) *Homosexuality: Research Implications for Public Policy*. Newbury Park, CA: Sage.
Simon, G. (forthcoming) Individual identity and group membership: some reflections on the politics of a postmodernist therapy. *Human Systems: Journal of Systemic Consultation and Management*.
Simons, S. (1991) Couple therapy with lesbians, in D. Hooper and W. Dryden (eds) *Couple Therapy: A Handbook*. Milton Keynes: Open University Press.
Simpson, M. (1992) Male impersonators. *Gay Times*, 167, August: 51–4.
Sinfield, A. (1994) *The Wilde Century: Effeminacy, Oscar Wilde and the Queer Movement*. London: Cassell.
Smith, J. (1988) Psychopathology, homosexuality and homophobia, in M. W. Ross (ed.) *The Treatment of Homosexuals with Mental Health Disorders*. New York: Harrington Park Press.
Smith, K. T. (1971) Homophobia: a tentative personality profile. *Psychological Reports*, 29: 1091–4.
Sontag, S. (1987) Notes on 'Camp', in *Against Interpretation*. London: Andre Deutsch.
Sophie, J. (1985) Stress, social network and sexual orientation identity change in women. *Dissertation Abstracts International*, 46, 949B (University Microfilms No. 85-10777).
Sophie, J. (1988) Internalized homophobia and lesbian identity, in E. Coleman (ed.) *Integrated Identity for Gay Men and Lesbians*. New York: Harrington Park Press.
Spinelli, E. (1989) *An Introduction to Phenomenological Psychology*. London: Sage.
Stacey, K. (1993) Exploring stories of lesbian experience in therapy: implications for therapists in a postmodern world. *Dulwich Centre Newsletter*, No. 2 Adelaide: 3–13.
Stall, R. and Wiley, J. (1988) A comparison of alcohol and drug patterns of homosexual and heterosexual men: the San Francisco men's health study. *Drug and Alcohol Dependence*, 22: 63–73.
Stein, T. S. (1988) Theoretical considerations in psychotherapy with gay men and

lesbians, in M. W. Ross (ed.) *The Treatment of Homosexuals with Mental Health Disorders*. New York: Harrington Park Press.
Stevens, C. T. (1993) Individuation and eros: finding my way, in R. H. Hopcke, K. L. Carrington and S. Wirth (eds) *Same Sex Love and the Path to Wholeness: Perspectives on Gay and Lesbian Psychological Development*. Boston, MA: Shambala.
Stubrin, J. P. (1994) *Sexualities and Homosexualities*. London: Karnac Books.
Tessina, T. (1989) *Gay Relationships: How to Find Them, How to Improve Them, How to Make Them Last*. Los Angeles, CA: Jeremy P. Tarcher Inc.
Thompson, R. (ed.) (1993) *Religion, Ethnicity, Sex Education: Exploring the Issues*. London: National Children's Bureau.
Tievsky, D. L. (1988) Homosexual clients and homophobic social workers. *Journal of Independent Social Work*, 2(3): 51–62.
Tinney, J. S. (1983) Interconnections. *Interracial Books for Children Bulletin*, 14, 3–4. New York: Council on Interracial Books for Children.
Tremble, B., Schneider, M. and Appathurai, C. (1989) Growing up gay or lesbian in a multicultural context, in G. Herdt (ed.) *Gay and Lesbian Youth*. New York: Haworth Press.
Trenchard, L. and Warren, H. (1984) *Something to Tell You*. London: London Gay Teenage Group.
Tripp, C. A. (1975) *The Homosexual Matrix*. New York: McGraw-Hill.
Troiden, R. R. (1979) Becoming homosexual: a model of gay identity acquisition. *Psychiatry*, 42(4): 362–73.
Ventura, L. A. (1983) 'Acceptance and maintenance of a lesbian identity', unpublished research paper University of Toledo. Quoted in P. A. Groves and L. A. Ventura, The lesbian coming out process: therapeutic considerations. *Personnel and Guidance Journal*, 8(1) November: 47–60.
Walsh, F. (1992) 'Cycle of oppression', unpublished training aid.
Weeks, J. (1985) *Sexuality and Its Discontents*. London: Routledge & Kegan Paul.
Weinberg, G. (1972) *Society and the Healthy Homosexual*. New York: St. Martin's Press.
Weinberg, M. S. and Williams, C. J. (1974) *Male Homosexuals: Their Problems and Adaptations*. New York: Oxford University Press.
Weinberg, T. (1978) On doing and being gay: Sexual behaviour and male self-identity. *Journal of Homosexuality*, 4: 143–56.
Weinrich J. D. and Williams, W. L. (1991) Strange customs, familiar lives: homosexualities in other cultures, in J. C. Gonsiorek and J. D. Weinrich (eds) *Homosexuality: Research Implications for Public Policy*. Newbury Park, CA: Sage Publications.
West, D. J. (1955) *Homosexuality*. London: Duckworth.
White, M. (1991) Deconstruction and therapy, *Experience Contradiction Narrative and Imagination*. Adelaide: Dulwich Centre Publications.
Woodman, N. J. and Lenna, H. R. (1980) *Counselling with Gay Men and Women: A Guide for Facilitating Positive Lifestyles*. San Francisco, CA: Jossey Bass.
Yalom, I. D. (1980) *Existential Psychotherapy*. New York: Basic Books.
Yalom, I. D. (1985) *The Theory and Practice of Group Psychotherapy*, 3rd edn. New York: Basic Books.
Young, V. (1995a) The menopause, in M. Jacobs (ed.) *The Care Guide: An Interdisciplinary Guide for the Caring Professions*. London: Mowbray.
Young, V. (1995b) *The Equality Complex: Lesbians in Therapy – a Guide to Anti-Oppressive Practice*. London: Cassell.

Index

abuse
　verbal/physical, 139–40, 145
　see also partner abuse
abusers, working with, 197
access to information/helplines, 71
adolescents, see young people (working with)
adoption and fostering, 128–9
affirmative therapy, see gay affirmative therapy
age of consent, 133–6
ageism, 152–5, 161, 163
agencies, 213–15
Agresti, A. A., 143
AIDS, 4–5, 70, 134, 136–7, 156, 202–3, 215
Albert Kennedy Trust, 129, 146, 213
Alcohol Concern, 216
alcohol misuse, 32, 58, 166–7
　attitudes, 179–80
　clinical implications, 177–8
　commitment of therapist, 178
　definitions/disclaimers, 170–1
　knowledge of therapist, 178–9
　model of use, 171–2
　principles of good practice, 180–7
　skills of therapist, 179
　substance use as issue, 172–7
　theory of counselling, 179
Alcoholics Anonymous, 171, 172, 183
Alcorn, K., 46

alienation, 77–8, 79, 161, 201
Allport, Gordon, 42, 43
ambisexual strategy, 79
American Psychiatric Association, 19–20
American Psychoanalytic Association, 21
American Psychological Association, 16
Amundson, J., 106
anger, 32, 73–4, 81
　projection of, 73–5
　see also partner abuse
anonymity problem, 15
anonymous artificial insemination by donor, 126
anonymous donor self-insemination, 126
anti-gay prejudice, 41–2, 50–1, 54
Arena 3 (magazine), 151
armed forces, 141
artificial insemination by donor, 126
Asch, A., 97
assertiveness training, 18
assessment, 34, 162
assimilation (coping strategy), 56
Association of Greater London Older Women (AGLOW), 152, 213
Association for Lesbian, Gay and Bisexual Psychologies, 27, 210–13
attitudes, 28–9, 70, 179–80
attraction to unavailable people, restricting (coping strategy), 63
authority (of therapist), 34–5
aversion therapy, 18

Index

awareness, HIV, 35–7
awareness of feelings, 31–2

Backman, C., 76
bargaining stage (Woodman–Lenna model), 71, 74–5
Barnes, M., 152, 157
Basic Instinct (film), 48
Bass, E., 152
Beard, J., 168
Beckett, E., 151
Begelman, D. A., 18
behaviour, homosexual, 11–12, 13
behaviour therapy, 18
Beiber, I., 14
beliefs, 28–9, 70
Bell, A. P., 57, 68, 132, 161
Bennett, K. C., 161
bereavement, 163–4
Bernard, D., 43
Bernstein, B., 143
Berzon, Betty, 29, 93
Bi Community News (magazine), 216
'Bible bingo', 201
bibliotherapy, 35, 57, 201
Bicon (conference), 99–100
Bifrost (magazine), 99
Bion, W., 166
biphobia, 4, 42, 57, 69
Bisexual Helpline, 213
bisexuality, 3–4, 12
    coming out, 69–70
    declassification of homosexuality, 1–2
    meeting others, 58, 90
black gay men, 165–6, 185–6, 214
Black Lesbian and Gay Helpline, 214
black lesbians, 154–5, 214
Blair, R., 17
Bland, L., 150
Bloomfield, K., 174, 176
Blumenfeld, W. J., 42, 44
Blumenstein, P., 92
Boden, R., 97–8
body–self/body impulses, 32–3
body image, 91–3, 94, 98–9
Boston Lesbian Psychologies Collective, 59
Boswell, J., 45, 200
Boxer, A. M., 132
Brand, P. A., 91
Bremner, J., 59
British Association for Counselling, 27, 50, 211

British Medical Association, 133
Buhrke, R. A., 25, 51
bullying, 135, 139–40, 145
Burbridge, M., 132, 140, 143
Burch, B., 109
Burgner, M., 167
Burke, M., 141
Burstow, B., 195
Burtle, V., 173

Cameron, Paul, 16
Caprio, F., 150
Capurro, Scott, 161
Card, C., 153
carers (potential homophobia), 71
Carl, Doug, 64, 104–5, 167
case examples, 6
    body image, 92–3
    coming out, 72–4
    disability, 99–100
    good practice (substance misuse), 180–2, 184–6
    internalized homophobia, 59–64
    older gay men, 162–7
    partner abuse, 191–3
    race/cross-cultural issues, 96–7
    religious/spirituality conflicts, 201, 202–6
    working with couples, 109–14
    working with young people, 136
Cass, Vivienne, 76
Cass model, 67, 76–82
Catalan, J., 159
causes, 14, 15
    ethics of, 16–19
Cayleff, S., 29, 52
Celluloid Closet, The (Russo), 48–9
ceremony and ritual, 202–6
change, 37–8, 155–6, 186–7
Channel Four programmes, 49, 152
Chapman, Diane, 150
childlessness, 129–30
children
    non-parental care, 129–30
    sexual abuse, 43, 138, 152
    see also children in single sex households; young people (working with)
Children Act (1989), 123, 125
children in single sex households, 116
    background, 117–19
    bringing children into relationship, 122–5

Index

common prejudices, 119–22
having children within relationship, 125–9
non-parental care, 129–30
sexual experimentation by, 144–5
uneasiness with (coping strategy), 63
Children's Society, 128
Chodorow, N., 150
Chou, S. P., 177
Christian 'conversion', 18–19
Christianity and homosexuality, 199, 200–2
Church of England, 103, 164
Churchill, W., 41
cinema (institutionalized homophobia), 48–9
city life, 69, 94
Clark, Don, 25–6, 29–34, 37, 39, 174
client
  empowerement, 197
  peer relationship with, 26–9, 33–4
clinical implications (substance misuse), 177–8
clinical manifestations of internalized homophobia), 58–64
clinical practice (institutionalized homophobia), 54
Clunis, D. G., 93
co-battery (partner abuse), 195
Cochrane, R., 174
Cody, J., 92
cognitive behavioural principles, 24
cognitive dissonance, 62
cognitive isolation, 135–6
cognitive restructuring, 56–7
Cohen, C., 39, 66
Cohen, E., 104
Cole, E., 153
Coleman, Eli, 67, 82, 139
Coleman model, 82–4
collaborative work, 106–7
coming out, 56, 57, 85, 136
  Cass model, 76–82
  Coleman model, 82–4
  definition, 66
  importance of, 67–71
  Woodman–Lenna model, 71–6
commitment, therapist, 178
community (lifestyle), 89–90
community resources, 213–16
community response (young people), 138–9

competition (barrier to intimacy), 93
confidentiality (guidelines), 146
conflict in family, 145–6
conflict management skills, 182
confrontation (coping strategy), 56
consciousness-raising, 33
conspiracy of silence, 45
consultation issues, 52–4
conversion/conversion therapy, 17–19, 37
Coordinated Management of Meaning, 111
coping strategies, 56–8, 62
core conditions, 24
  of respect, 2, 26–9
cottaging, 43, 53, 95
counselling
  assessment, 162
  theory, 25, 179
  Woodman–Lenna model, 28, 53, 67, 71–6, 144
counsellors, 6
  training, 50–2
counter-transference, 39, 71
couple therapy, 167
couples (working with)
  collaborative work, 106–7
  final reflections, 114–15
  generalisations/diversity, 101–2
  presenting for therapy, 107–14
  relationship choices, 102–6
couples counselling, 168, 197–8
Coyle, A., 1, 33, 58, 133
Crain, W. C., 51
Cramer, D. W., 143–4
Criminal Justice Act (1994), 133, 141, 194
Cromwell, A., 97
Cronin, D. M., 68
cross-cultural issues, 95–7
cross-dressing, 136
cross-sex grid, 20
cultural identity, 3–4, 48
cultural values, 96
culture
  cross-cultural issues, 95–7
  denial of, 45
  differences, 52, 165–6
  respect for, 27–8
cures, 1, 14, 15, 143, 172
  ethics of, 16–19
custody battles, 122–3

D'Aguelli, A. R., 94–5
Dank, B. M., 83
Davis, L., 152
Davison, G. C., 17, 18, 37
de Monteflores, Carmen, 56, 67
Deaf Lesbian and Gay Groups, 214
death
　bereavement, 163–4
　suicide, 32, 36, 58, 75, 135, 137–8, 201
declassification of homosexuality, 1–2
defence mechanisms, 58–63, 72–3, 77, 82
defined public spaces, 45–6
definitions, 6
　of homophobia, 41–2
　of older lesbians, 149–50
　of sexuality, 11–13
　substance/alcohol misuse, 170–1
denial
　of culture, 45
　as defence mechanism, 58, 62–3, 72, 77
　of partner abuse, 196–7
　of popular strength, 45
　of self-labelling, 46
　stage (Woodman–Lenna model), 71–3
Department of Health and Human Services Task Force on Suicide, 135
dependency assessment (substance misuse), 184–5
depression, 32, 58, 135
　stage (Woodman–Lenna), 71, 75–6
developmental lag (Coleman model), 83, 84, 139
developmental stages, 25, 51
Di Clemente, C. C., 186
Diagnostic Statistical Manual, 19–20
Diamond, D. L., 173
Dignity in the USA, 202
disability, 70–1, 97–100, 154, 155
disclosure, see coming out; self-disclosure
discovery, fear of, 59
discrimination, 43, 97, 153, 155
　institutionalized homophobia, 42, 44–54
'disease model', 172, 183
'dispiritation', 32, 93
dissonance reduction, 62
Diva (magazine), 216

diversity/generalisations, 101–2
Dollimore, J., 20
domestic violence, see partner abuse
Domestic Violence Intervention projects, 216
Dörner, Gunter, 16
Dowrick, Stephanie, 205
drag queens, 136
Driggs, J. H., 93
drug misuse, 32
　see also substance misuse
Duffy, Maureen, 150

Eckhart, Meister, 201
education, 47–8, 134, 139–40
educative function (therapist), 35–7
effeminacy, 43, 74, 92, 121, 136
ego-dystonic homosexuality, 20
ego-syntonic homosexuality, 62
ego defence mechanisms, 58, 72
Ehrhardt, A. A., 82
eight stages of development (Erikson), 25, 51, 67
Elfin Moses, A., 90, 98
Ellis, M. L., 22
emotion, awareness of, 31–2
emotional intimacy, 93–4
emotional isolation, 135
employment, 49–50, 140–2
empowerment, 151, 154, 197
Epstein, D., 140
Erikson, E., 25, 51, 67, 205
Ernst, S., 151
erotophobia, 64
Espin, O. M., 95, 96
ethics, 37–8
　of causes/cures, 16–19
　of touching, 33
　of treatment, 17–18
ethnic diversity, 3, 165–6
Etnyre, W. S., 91, 92
Eurocentrism, 96, 97
ex-partners (reaction to gay parenting), 122–3
exploration stage (Coleman model), 83

Fairlie, J., 157
Falco, Kristine L., 174
Family and Friends of Lesbians and Gays (FFLAG), 143, 147, 214
family issues, 142–6
Farley, N., 189

Index

Fashanu, Justin, 69
Fay, R. E., 132
fear of discovery, 59
fear of homosexuality, see homophobia
fear of over-visibility, 45
feelings, awareness of, 31–2
feminism, 35, 151, 156, 168
femininity, 20, 92
Fifield, L., 173
Fine, M., 97
Finn, S. E., 93
first relationships, 84
Forstein, M., 50, 55
Fortunato, 201
fostering and adoption, 128–9
Foucault, M., 104
Fox, M., 201
Frank, J., 161
Frankie and Johnnie (film), 48
Frankl, Viktor, 203, 205
Freud, S., 19, 20, 21, 23, 25, 51, 79, 168
Freudianism, 121
Freund, K. W., 15, 42
Friedman, R. C., 168
Friends and Families of Lesbians and Gays (FFLAG), 143, 147, 214
friendship (role), 168
Fromm, E., 205
future developments, 7

gay affirmative therapy, 19, 21, 84
  core conditions, 2, 24, 26–9
  ethical issues, 37–8
  finding a therapist, 27, 210–12
  guidelines, 30–5
  for older lesbians, 153–5
  model development, 24–5
  sexual orientation of therapist, 38–9
  therapist as educator, 35–7
  training, 1–2, 29–30
Gay and Lesbian Legal Advice, 214
gay bashing, 43, 193
gay community, 89–90
gay identity, 13, 57
Gay Liberation Front, 70
gay men
  coming out, see coming out
  declassification policy, 1–2
  defining sexuality, 6, 11–13
  generation issues (options), 125–9
  support systems, 33, 69, 90

gay men, older (working with)
  assessment, 162
  case examples, 162–7
  conclusions, 167–9
  therapy, 159–62
gay pride, 38, 45–6, 62
Gay Pride March, 38, 45–6
Gay Scotland (magazine), 216
gay support systems, 33, 69, 90
Gay Switchboard, 49, 214
Gay Times, 31, 49, 214, 216
gay villages, 45
Gay's the Word Bookshop, 217
Gebhard, P. H., 12
'Gemma', 99
gender, 20, 21
  in coming out process, 68
  identity, see identity
  partner abuse (comparisons), 191–2
  roles, 44, 78
generalisation/diversity, 101–2
genital stages (Freud), 25, 51
ghettoization (coping strategy), 56
Gilroy, B., 154
'Glad to be Gay' anthem, 81
Glaser, C., 201
Glickauf-Hughes, C., 168
God (spirituality conflicts), 199–202, 204, 205, 206
Golombok, S., 121
Gonsiorek, J. C., 12, 15, 17, 20, 55, 64, 90, 139
good practice, principles of (alcohol and substance misuse), 180–7
Goode, E., 132
Goodison, L., 151
Grace, J., 67, 83, 139
Gramick, J., 52
Grau, G., 21
Greasley, P., 49–50
Green, D., 93
Green, R., 121
Greene, B., 153
Groves, P. A., 68
guidelines, 30–5, 146–7
guilt, 34, 75, 83
Gutierrez, F. J., 152, 153, 159

Haber, L., 132
habituation to homosexuality, 58
Haddith: An-Nasa'i, 200
Haldeman, D. C., 17, 18, 19
Hall, Marny, 27, 109, 112

Hall, Radclyffe, 150
Hall Carpenter Archives, 160
Hall Carpenter Archives/Lesbian History Group, 151, 152
'Halloween Letter' (1986), 200
Hammond, Nancy, 196
Hanley-Hackenbruck, P., 66, 70
harassment, 139–40, 145
harm
  assessment (substance misuse), 184–5
  self-harm, 58, 75, 135, 145, 184
Harriman, R. E., 42
Harris, S., 140
Hart, M., 20
Hawkins, R., 52
Hawxhurst, Donna M., 198
Heather, N., 172
Hedblom, J. H., 132
Helfand, K. L., 162
helplines, 71, 213–15
Hemmings, D., 151
Hencker, F. O., 98
Hepburn, G., 152, 153
Herek, G. M., 16, 41, 43–4, 64, 153
heterophobia, 62
heterosexism, 4, 16, 22, 24, 30, 38–9, 153, 176
  see also homophobia and heterosexism
heterosexual assertiveness training, 18
heterosexual questionnaire, 209
heterosexual sex (lesbian mothers), 127
heterosexual therapist, 38–9
heterosexual unions, children from previous, 122, 125
heterosexuality, 15–16, 62
  partner abuse and, 191–3
Hetrick, E. S., 75, 134, 135, 138
Hetrick-Martin Institute, 134
Hidden Holocaust, The (Grau), 21
Hildebrand, H. P., 167
Hillin, A., 59–61
historical overview
  defining sexuality, 11–13
  research, 13–16
  researchers, 16–19
  therapy-homosexuality relationship, 19–22
HIV, 4–5, 134, 136–7, 163–4, 168, 204
  awareness, 35–7
Hocquenghem, Guy, 20
Holtzen, D. W., 143
homoerotophobia, 41

homonegativism, 41
homophobe (a portrait), 44
homophobia and heterosexism, 4, 16, 24, 25, 28–30, 65, 67, 146, 147
  definitions, 41–2
  functions of prejudice, 42–4
  institutionalized homophobia, 44–6
  institutionalized homophobia in society, 46–50
  institutionalized homophobia within mental health professions, 50–4
  internalized homophobia, 42, 54–64
homophobia and partner abuse, 193
homosexism, 41, 94
homosexophobia, 41
homosexual behaviour, 11–12, 13
homosexual identity, 11, 13
homosexuality
  Christianity and, 200–2
  declassification, 1–2
  future developments, 7
  study aims/limitation, 2–5
  terms/definition, 6
  therapy and (historical overview), 11–23
  see also bisexuality; gay men; lesbian women
Hooker, Evelyn A., 20
hormone replacement therapy, 157
Hudson, Rock, 103
Hudson, W. W., 41
Human Fertilisation and Embryology Authority, 215
humanistic model, 2, 25

Iasenza, S., 29–30
identification with aggressor, 59, 63
identity, 131, 132
  acceptance (Cass model), 80–1
  comparison (Cass model), 77–9
  confusion (Cass model), 76–7
  confusion (Woodman–Lenna model), 71, 73–4
  development/formation, 67
  homosexual, 11, 13
  integration (Coleman model), 84
  label, 57
  negative, 57
  pride (Cass model), 81
  synthesis (Cass model), 81–2
  see also self-identity
indecent assault, 194
Institute of Marital Studies, 167

Institute for the Protection of Lesbian and Gay Youth, 134
Institute for the Study of Drug Dependence, 216
institutionalized heterosexism, 38
institutionalized homophobia, 42, 44–6
 in society, 46–50
 within mental health professions, 50–4
integrative model, 186
interactionist model, 76–82
interest groups, 49
internalized ageism, 163
internalized homophobia, 42, 54–64, 80, 104, 135, 142, 160, 164–5, 176, 193
International Classification of Diseases (ICD), 1, 19
intimacy, emotional, 93–4
Intimacy and Solitude (Dowrick), 205
invisibility, 32, 74, 94, 140
 consequences of, 102–4
Iraneus, Saint, 200
Isay, R. A., 20–1, 25, 30–1, 55, 80, 83
Isensee, R., 93
Islam, 199, 200
isolation, 134–6, 138–9, 140

Jay, K., 68, 83
Jeffreys, S., 155
jokes, anti-gay, 31, 32, 43
Jourard, S., 32, 93
Journal of Studies on Alcohol, 173
Judaism, 200
Jung, C. J., 205

Kenric, 151
Khambatta, A., 153, 154–5
Kimmel, D. C., 67
Kinsey Report (1947), 11, 12, 17, 45, 54, 145
Kinsey Report (1953), 11, 132
Kippax, S., 137
Kirsch, J. A. W., 13
Kitzinger, C., 20, 106–7, 155
Klaich, D., 150
Klassen, A. D., 41
Klein, C., 151
knowledge (therapist), 178–9
known donor self-insemination, 127–8
Krajeski, J. P., 16, 18, 25
Kübler-Ross, E., 71
Kus, R. J., 35

labelling, 46, 58, 104
Lago, C., 97
Langevin, R., 42
Langley, Esme, 150
language and meaning, 182–3, 206
Lavender Couch, The (Hall), 27
Le Vay, Simon, 17
Lee, J. A., 159
legislation, 17, 47, 123, 125, 133, 141, 194
Lehne, G. K., 41
leisure (institutionalized homophobia), 48–9
Lendrum, S., 164
Lenna, H. R., 28, 53, 67, 71–6, 144
Lesbian and Gay Bereavement Project, 214
Lesbian and Gay Christian Movement, 202, 214
Lesbian and Gay Employment Rights, 49
Lesbian and Gay Foster and Adoptive Parents Network, 214
Lesbian Information Service, 214
lesbian women
 coming out, *see* coming out
 declassification policy, 1–2
 defining sexuality, 6, 11–13
 generation issues (options), 125–8
 mothers (previous heterosexual unions), 122
 support systems, 33, 69, 90
lesbian women, older (working with)
 definitions, 149–50
 developing affirmative therapy approach, 153–5
 formation of lesbian identity, 150–1
 resources, 152–3
 therapy, 151–2
 therapy issues, 155–8
Levitt, E. E., 41
Lewes, K., 168
Lewis, R. A., 93
lifestyles, 27–8, 89–90, 94–5, 185–6
Limentani, A., 167
Lindenfield, G., 32
Lisuride (drug), 16
local authority care, 145–6
Local Government Act (1988), 134
Local Government Act (1990), 47
locale factor (coming out), 69
Lohrenz, L., 173
London Lesbian and Gay Switchboard, 214

London Lesbian and Gay Teenage
    Group, 75
loss, mid-life (older lesbians), 156–8
Loulan, J., 156

MacDonald, B., 153–4
McDonald, G. J., 67
McKirnan, D. J., 173, 174, 175
McLellan, B., 155
McNeil, John, 201, 202
magazines, 216
Manosevitz, M., 132
'map' (single sex parenting), 118–19
Maple, N., 152, 157
Margolies, L., 56, 58–9, 62–4
Marie (1992), 155
Martin, A. D., 75, 134, 135, 138
masculinity, 20, 43, 92, 191–2, 194
Mason-John, V., 153, 154–5
Masson, J., 20
May, R., 205
Maylon, A., 25
Mays, V. M., 96
meaning and language, 182–3, 206
medical model, 1, 14, 15, 21, 172
    ethics of, 16–19
meeting people, 58, 90
Mencher, J., 109
menopause, 156–8
mental health professions, 50–4
Messing, A. E., 53
methodology flaws, 14–16
Metropolitan Community Church, 202
Meyer, J. K., 12
Microcosm, The (Duffy), 150
mid-life transition, 156–8
Midanik, L., 174
MIND, 152, 211
Minorities Research Group, 151
Minton, H., 67
Money, J., 82
'moral crusader', 77
Morrow, Susan L., 198
Moses, A., 52
Mosher, D. L., 39
motivation (of researchers), 16–17

Narcotics Anonymous, 171, 172
Nardi, Peter, 173
National AIDS Helpline, 215
National Children's Bureau, 133
National Friend, 156, 215
National Health Service, 16, 159

nature–nurture theory, 13–14
Navratilova, Martina, 48, 103
Nazism, 21 *bis*
negative effects of therapy, 37–8
negative feelings, 36–7, 44, 54–64
negative identity (avoiding), 57
negative reactions (of homophobe), 44
negative stereotypes, 44, 46, 56
negative symbolism, 46
Neild, S., 152, 153
Neisen, J. H., 41
neurosurgery, 17
new relationships, children in, 124
newspapers, 216
non-gay specialist organizations, 215–16
non-parental child care, 129–30
nurture–nature theories, 13–14

Oberndorf, Clarence, 21
occupational choice (of young people), 141–2
O'Connor, N., 22, 150, 168
Oedipal theory, 20
older gay men, *see* gay men, older (working with)
older lesbian women, *see* lesbian women, older (working with)
Older Lesbians Conference, 152
openness, aversion to (barrier to intimacy), 93
oppression, 20, 31–2, 34, 43, 92
    cycle of, 46–7, 59, 60–1
    of lesbians, 150, 151, 153
Orbach, S., 21
Otitojou, Femi, 154
over-visibility (single parenting), 124

paedophilia, 43, 138
parasuicide, 137–8
parenting (lesbian and gay), 63, 116
    background, 117–19
    bringing children into same sex relationships, 122–5
    common prejudices, 119–22
    having children within same sex relationships, 125–9
    non-parental child care, 129–30
    parents and family issues, 142–6
Parmar, P., 154
partner abuse
    co-battery, 195
    comparisons with heterosexual problems, 191–3

couples counselling, 197–8
definitions/terms, 188–90
implications for therapists, 195–7
rape and sexual assault, 194–5
sado-masochism, 193–4
patriarchy, 43
Pearce, W. B., 111
Pearson, R., 152, 153
peripheral hormone injections, 18
Perkins, R., 20, 155
personal innocence strategy, 79
personal integrity, respect for, 26–7
personality development, 25, 51
Peterson, P. L., 173, 174, 175
Phillips, A., 153, 155, 157
physical appearance, 91–3, 94
physical attack, 43
physical contact, 32–3
physical harassment, 139–40, 145
physical impairment (coming out process), 70–1
Pines, M., 162
Pink Paper, The, 71, 216
plethysmograph, 15
Plummer, K., 83
police (employment in), 141
police arrest records, 43
political change, 155–6
political identity (of bisexuality), 3–4
power, 82, 191, 192, 193
  of therapist, 20, 26, 34
pre-coming out stage (Coleman model), 82–3
Pregnancy Advisory Service, 126, 215
prejudice, 153
  anti-gay, 41–2, 50–1, 54
  functions of, 42–4
  institutionalized homophobia, 42, 44–54
  internalized homophobia, 42, 54–64
  of single sex parenting, 116, 119–22, 124
primary technique, 205–6
Prochaska, J. O., 186
Project for Advice, Counselling and Education (PACE), 215
Project Sigma, 176
projection (defence mechanism), 59, 62, 72
projection of anger, 73–5
promiscuity, 46, 135
psychoanalysis, 14, 18, 20–2, 25

psychodynamic model, 2, 24, 25, 59, 159, 162, 163
psychopathology, 22
psychotherapy, 25, 50, 179, 199
  with older gay men, 159–63, 167
  with older lesbians, 151–2
psychospiritual growth, 199, 202, 204–5
public spaces, defined, 45–6

Quakers, 200
quality of therapy, 71
Queer in America (Signorile), 49
queer bashing, 43, 193
questionnaires, 14, 15, 16, 209

Rabin, J., 53
race factor, 3, 68–9, 95–7
racism, 154–5
Rakusen, J., 153, 155, 157
Ramsey, G. V., 132
rape (partner abuse), 194–5
Raphael, B., 164
Ratigan, Bernard, 79
rationalization (defence mechanism), 59, 62, 72
Ratzinger, Cardinal, 200
Raymond, D., 42
reaction formation, 58, 62, 140
REGARD, 99, 215
Reiss, B. F., 20
relationship choices, 102–6
relationships (after coming out), 84
relationships, people in (working with)
  collaborative work, 106–7
  final reflection/conclusion, 114–15
  generalisations/diversity, 101–2
  presenting for therapy, 107–14
  relationship choices, 102–6
religious/spirituality conflicts, 34, 199, 207
  Christian 'conversion', 18–19
  Christianity and homosexuality, 200–2
  ritual and ceremony, 202–6
religious exorcism/prayer, 18
repression (defence mechanism), 72
research methods, 13–16
researchers, 16–19
residential care, 145–6
resources, 152–3, 213–16
respect, 2, 25, 26–9
retraining, 29–30
Rich, C., 153–4

Ricketts, W. A., 41
ritual and ceremony, 202–6
Rivers, Ian, 47, 134, 135, 139
Roach, A. J., 143–4
Roberts, J., 162
Robertson, I., 172
Robins, E., 58, 173
Robinson, G., 138
Rochlin, M., 209
Rogers, C., 24, 39, 205
'role distancing', 78
role models, 48, 93
  for children, 120–1, 124, 129
  coming out, 75, 80, 84
  gay affirmative model, 33, 35, 39
  gay relationships, 103, 104, 113
  for young people, 136, 139, 142
Ross, M. W., 159
Ross-Reynolds, G., 132
Rothblum, E. D., 135, 153
Rowe, Dorothy, 205
Rudolph, J. R., 55, 90
rural life, 94–5
Ruse, M., 14, 19
Russell, J., 33
Russo, Vito, 48–9
Ruszczynski, S., 167
Rutter, P., 33
Ryan, J., 22, 150, 157, 168

sado-masochism, 37, 193–4
safer sex behaviour, 35–7, 137, 176
Saghir, M. T., 58, 173
Sanderson, T., 93
Sandmaier, M., 173
Sang, B., 150, 153
Sappho, 151
Savin-Williams, R. C., 131
school/education, 47–8, 134, 139–40
Schultz, S. J., 67
Schwartz, P., 92
Secord, P. F., 76
self-alienation, 161, 201
self-assessment, 34
self-awareness, 205–6
self-blame (partner abuse), 196–7
self-definition, 6, 11, 133, 151, 170
self-disclosure, 15, 39, 57, 93–4, 96
self-empowerment, 151, 154
self-esteem, 176, 177
  coming out and, 75, 79–80, 82–3
  gay affirmative therapy, 26, 32, 36–8
  homophobia and, 43, 57

  of single people, 90, 92
  of young people, 133–8 *passim*, 142–3
self-harm, 58, 75, 135, 145, 184
self-hate, 79, 80, 177, 206
self-help, 93, 151, 217–21
self-identity, 6, 12, 57, 79, 132–3, 156
self-image, 91, 95, 193
self-insemination, 126–7
self-labelling, 46, 58
sensory impairment (coming out process), 70–1
Sergios, P., 92
sexism, 153
sexual abuse (of children), 43, 138, 152
sexual assault (partner abuse), 194–5
sexual identity, 131, 132
sexual orientation, 131, 132
  of client (respect for), 26
  of therapist, 38–9
sexual preferences, substance use and, 182–3
sexual variation, extent of (coming out process), 69–70
sexuality
  defining, 11–13
  gender and, 20, 21
  see also bisexuality; gay men; heterosexuality; homosexuality; lesbian women
Shakespeare, T., 98
shame, 34, 41, 75, 83
Shapiro, J., 153
Shepherd, S., 160
Shernoff, M., 35–7, 137
Shields, S. A., 42
Shively, M. D., 57
short-term relationships, 63–4
Sigma project, 176
Signorile, Michelangelo, 49
Silberstein, L., 92
silence, conspiracy of, 45
silence (value/role), 206
Silverstein, C., 16, 17, 37, 162
Simon, G., 107, 113–14
Simpson, Mark, 31
Sinfield, Alan, 20, 22, 31, 92, 121
single people (working with)
  body image, 91–3
  community, 89–90
  disability, 97–100
  emotional intimacy, 93–4
  meeting others, 90

race and cross-cultural issues, 95–7
rural lesbian/gay lives, 94–5
single sex parents, *see* parenting (lesbian and gay)
skills (therapist), 179
Smith, J., 58
Smith, K. T., 41
Socarides, Charles, 16
social alienation, 77–8, 79
social change, 155–6
social control, 200
social isolation, 134–5
social learning theory, 18, 172, 175
social services (role), 145–6
social space, 45–6
socialization process, 29, 55, 68, 80, 83, 91–2
society, 44–50, 147
Society of Friends, 200
Sontag, S., 160
Sophie, J., 39, 56–7, 58
special case strategy, 79
special interest groups, 49
specialization (coping strategy), 56
Spinelli, E., 163
spirituality, *see* religious/spirituality conflicts
sports, 48
Stacey, Kathleen, 114
Stall, R., 173, 175
Stein, Gertrude, 103
Stein, T. S., 39, 66
stereotypes, 153
  coming out and, 74, 78
  gay affirmative therapy model, 24, 31, 33
  homophobia and, 43, 44, 46, 48–50, 56
  self-esteem and, 43, 83, 90, 92, 136
Stevens, C. T., 153
Stewart, Elizabeth, 202
stigmatization, 41–65, 67, 137–8, 139
Stonewall group, 141
'strange loop' (relationships), 111–12
Straub (in Burtle), 173
Stubrin, J. P., 168
sublimation (defence mechanism), 72–3
substance misuse
  attitudes, 179–80
  clinical implications, 177–8
  definitions/disclaimers, 170–1
  models of use, 171–2
  principles of good practice, 180–7

substance use as issue, 172–7
theories of counselling, 179
therapist skills, 178–9
suicide, 32, 36, 58, 75, 135, 137–8, 201
supervision, 52–4
suppression (defence mechanism), 72–3
survivor guilt, 156, 163
symbolism, negative, 46
Syme, G., 164

Tavistock Clinic, 167
television (institutionalized homophobia), 48–9
temporary identity strategy, 79
Terrence Higgins Trust, 54
Tessina, T., 93
theatre (institutionalized homophobia), 48–9
therapists, 6
  authority of, 34–5
  commitment, 178
  core conditions, 2, 24, 26–9
  as educator, 35–7
  ethical issues, 37–8
  guidelines, 30–5, 146–7
  implications for (of partner abuse), 195–7
  knowledge, 178–9
  leaflet on finding, 27, 210–12
  sexual orientation, 38–9
  skills, 179
  supervision/consultation, 52–4
  see also counsellors
therapy
  historical overview, 11–23
  quality of, 71
  reasons for presenting for, 107–14
  relationship to homosexuality, 19–22
  see also counselling
Thompson, J., 97
Thompson, N. L., 161
Thompson, R., 200
'Three Essays on the Theory of Sexuality' (Freud), 20
Tievsky, D. L., 52
Tinney, J. S., 44
Toklas, Alice B., 103
Toksvig, Sandy, 103
touch (therapeutic value), 32–3
training, 1–2, 22, 29–30, 50–2
transactional analysis, 181–2
transference, 36–7, 39, 71
transtheoretical therapy, 186

treatment, 1, 14, 145, 172
  ethics of, 17–18
Tremble, B., 95–6
Trenchard, L., 75, 135, 137, 142, 145
'trigger comments', 183
Troiden, R. R., 67, 68
'Twelve-Steps' philosophy, 171

Valentino, Rudolph, 103
value systems, 33–4, 78
Ventura, L. A., 68
verbal harassment, 139–40
verbal rejection, 43
violence
  gay bashing, 43, 193
  physical harassment, 139–40, 145
  self-harm, 58, 75, 135, 145, 184
  suicide, 32, 36, 58, 75, 135, 137–8, 201
  see also partner abuse
Violence Prevention Programme, 216
visibility/invisibility, 32, 45, 74, 94, 102–4, 140
Voice, The (newspaper), 69

Wallis, M., 160
Walsh, Fran, 46–7
Walters, J., 132, 140, 143
Warren, H., 75, 135, 137, 142, 145
Weeks, J., 13, 20
Weinberg, G., 41, 43
Weinberg, M. S., 18, 57, 68, 132, 161

Weinberg, T., 68
Weinrich, J. D., 12, 13, 15
Well of Loneliness, The (Hall), 150
West, D. J., 161
White, M., 102
wider system questions, 113–14
Wilde Century, The (Sinfield), 92, 121
Wiley, J., 173, 175
Williams, C. J., 18
Williams, W. L., 13
Wilsnack, S. C., 173
Women Like Us (Channel Four), 152
Women's Health, 215
Women's Support Service, 216
Woodman, N. J. (Woodman–Lenna model), 28, 53, 67, 71–6, 144
work issues, 140–2
World Health Organization, 19

xenophobia, 64

Yalom, I. D., 161, 163
Young, A., 68, 83
Young, V., 151, 157
young people (working with), 131–2, 148
  age of consent, 133–6
  guidelines for therapists, 146–7
  lesbian and gay community, 138–9
  parent and family issues, 142–6
  self-esteem issues, 136–8
  work and employment, 140–2